Preventing
Cancer

PREVENTING CANCER

Dr. Elizabeth Whelan

PREFACE BY PHILIP COLE, M.D.
HARVARD SCHOOL OF PUBLIC HEALTH

W · W · NORTON & COMPANY · INC ·
NEW YORK

Portions of Chapter 11 (specifically, that dealing with saccharin) originally appeared in *Across the Board*, published by the Conference Board, in June, 1977.

Portions of Chapter 12 originally appeared in *Harper's Bazaar*.

Library of Congress Cataloging in Publication Data

Whelan, Elizabeth M
    Preventing cancer.

    Bibliography: p.
    Includes index.
    1. Cancer—Prevention.   2. Carcinogenesis.
I. Title.
RC268.W53   616.9′94′05   77–26682
ISBN 0–393–06431–X

1 2 3 4 5 6 7 8 9 0

For *Christine*

CONTENTS

8 *Contents*

"Out of a Hundred Diseases, Fifty
Are Caused by Our Own Faults,
Forty by Our Carelessness."
Paolo Mantegazza

PREFACE

About a hundred and twenty-five years ago humans began to use science to prevent disease and not just to treat it. The first efforts were directed against the greatest foes. These were the infectious diseases, especially the great epidemic diseases of antiquity: plague, cholera, typhoid fever and typhus, malaria and yellow fever and tuberculosis. Prior to their being controlled, these diseases had imposed a severe burden of mortality on the human race. Moreover, there was very little that a person could do to lower his or her chances of developing one of them. Methods for eliminating these diseases had to be based almost exclusively on environmental control, not on the actions of individuals. With the advent of the "sanitary revolution," about seventy-five years ago, such methods became available and the epidemic diseases as well as many others were largely eradicated.

About thirty years ago, the science of disease prevention, epidemiology, was reborn and redirected. Now, the target was another great scourge, arteriosclerosis. Ateriosclerosis, or hardening of the arteries, causes many adverse effects, the most important being heart attacks and strokes. Here, too, the tide has been turned and great progress made. Although the reasons are not yet known with certainty, deaths from heart attack and stroke are declining in the United States. But whatever the reasons may be, they do *not* involve environmental control. The decline is due to personal changes in behavior: reduced smoking, reduced consumption of saturated fats, better control of diabetes and of hypertension and, perhaps, an increase in regular exercise. The lesson is clear: with respect to arteriosclerosis, each person is largely in control of his or her own fate.

About fifteen years ago, during the administration of President

Johnson, the People of the United States began an organized attack on cancer: the National Program for the Conquest of Heart Disease, Cancer, and Stroke. In 1971 the battle against cancer was rejoined with the start of the National Cancer Program. As yet the progress has been slow, almost imperceptible. But, we should appreciate that cancer has been attacked at its roots, at its causes, for less than twenty years. Moreover, cancer is a host of diseases, mostly different from one another in their causes. Thus, patience is necessary, but we can take comfort from the lessons of history which tell us that we will win. But while being patient, it is still reasonable to ask what can be done now. Can we see any glimmer of the direction in which to march? Will cancer be controlled by further sanitizing the environment or does individual behavior hold the key? The answer is: for cancer control *both* environmental changes and individual action will be required. In fact, even now a person can do a great deal to lower his or her cancer risk by using the information available regarding its causes. This book will show you what can be done.

The major purpose of Dr. Whelan's book is to describe what you can do and what you can teach your children to do to avoid cancer. The bases for the preventive measures are rational and are well described. The book tells how the measures follow, in a logical way, from existing knowledge of the causes of cancer. This is true even of cancers for which there is only a rough idea of causes. Of course, there can be no guarantee of protection against cancer. But, I would estimate that by following Dr. Whelan's recommendations a young man can lower his risk by at least 40 percent compared to the average, and a young woman by at least 25 percent.

This book also achieves a second important purpose. It provides a large and well-integrated body of accurate information on cancer. This will permit the reader to evaluate effectively the barrage of cancer-related items which appears almost daily in the news media. The implications of these items, usually difficult to perceive, should be clearer after reading this book. In addition, the news media are often inaccurate and this, too, will be more readily apparent.

Quite in passing, this book achieves a third and fascinating objective: it tells the story of cancer in our era, the era of the beginning of the conquest. In so doing, it provides a perspective which makes us indifferent to the doomsayers who claim, erroneously, that cancer is becoming epidemic in the United States. And, this perspective also helps us to tolerate the hopeless optimists for whom "breakthroughs" are a daily occurrence and the conquest imminent. As a bonus, the story is told in the clear, unemotional, and accurate prose of a woman who is herself a public health professional. Thus, Dr. Whelan's messages are explicit: The fight against cancer goes well but slowly. Control will come about from prevention much more than from cure. If we wish to avoid the disease, each of us must do what he or she can to minimize exposure to its known and suspected causes.

Philip Cole, M.D., Dr.P.H.

Associate Professor of Epidemiology
Harvard School of Public Health
Boston

Consultant in Epidemiology
International Agency for Research on Cancer
Lyon, France

INTRODUCTION

When I told a neighbor that I was writing a book entitled *Preventing Cancer*, she scoffed and said, "What are you going to tell them to do? Give up eating, drinking, and breathing?

"From what you hear," she went on, "everything these days causes cancer. The stuff they put in our food; the air we breathe; cigarettes; even plastic wrap and toothpaste. I say, 'Forget all of it.' It's a game of chance. You can't influence whether or not your number is going to come up. So just tune out, give in, and get on with your life."

Many Americans have come to accept the prevailing view that we are in the grip of an industrially caused cancer epidemic, surrounded by a sea of carcinogens, at the mercy of an array of noxious chemicals. Some, like my neighbor, believing that cancer threats are numerous and elusive, have become resigned, assuming an "oh-the-hell-with-it" attitude. Others are protesting what they believe to be a highly undesirable side effect of modern technology, demanding that we free ourselves from all "cancer-causing chemicals." Both groups have lost perspective. *Preventing Cancer* is an attempt to regain a proper perspective about what causes human cancer.

The book is based on four major premises. *First*, we do know a great deal about the causes of this varied group of diseases called cancer. Cancer is not, as Sir Winston Churchill described Russia in 1939, "a riddle wrapped in a mystery inside an enigma." Certainly there are many questions yet to be answered. But right now, there are ways of minimizing your chances of being a cancer victim. Indeed, *by following the advice in this book, you will, on the average, reduce your chances of developing cancer by some 20 to 50 percent or more*. Obviously, the percentage by which your probability of cancer is reduced by the recommendations here will be greatly influenced by your current age and previous exposures to cancer-promoting factors, a child of ten or younger benefiting most, a sixty-year-old with a long history of, for example, cigarette smoking, benefiting least. But even in his latter case, the counsel in *Preventing Cancer,* if followed carefully, should offer some protection from the disease. It should go without saying that no set of guidelines can offer you complete protection from all forms of cancer. What we are dealing with here are the means of considerably reducing your odds of developing some forms of the disease.

The emphasis here will be on primary, as opposed to secondary prevention, that is, ways you can avoid cancer before it begins, rather than means of detecting and curing it.

Second, there is a clear distinction between the factors known to increase human cancer risk and those which are at most hypothetical or merely suspected cancer hazards. The failure to make this distinction is the primary reason so many people today have lost perspective about cancer causation.

It's possible that anything, including strawberries, seawater, or felt-tip pens could cause cancer. It is virtually impossible to prove that these items are not involved in carcinogenesis. Of course, there is absolutely no solid evidence to suggest that they are. On the other hand, we do have an overwhelming amount of information indicating that some chemicals and behavior patterns *do* significantly increase one's risk of developing various forms of human cancer.

Given that the topic we're dealing with is a highly emotional one, it is relatively easy to call attention to a hypothetical risk. When it comes to cancer, people are both nervous and gullible. If I called a newspaper reporter and said that, in my professional judgment, it was the minute but regular ingestion of the glue on the back of American postage stamps which was responsible for our country's relatively high rate of colon cancer, I would probably stimulate at least one story on the subject. If I got one or two of my colleagues to second this opinion, and submitted a report about the toxic effect of postage stamp glue on Swiss white mice, my view would probably make headlines.

This is the type of material which makes news, whether or not it is supported by scientific data.

The cancer risk factors I'll describe in this book under the heading "known" are those which have been shown in professionally planned studies to increase the risk of malignant growths in human beings.

The three hypothetical risk factors discussed in Chapters 11, 12, and 13 which are included only for the purpose of comparison and to alleviate any concerns that you might now have about them, are those which have never been shown to cause cancer in human beings in the manner we now use them. The designation of these three topics as hypothetical risk factors does not necessarily mean that they never pose any problems under any circumstances. The categorization here is limited to cancer causation.

Of course, you can never rule out the possibility that some hypothetical risk factors may someday be proven to be real ones. But again, the same could be said about strawberries, seawater, and felt-tip pens. In terms of making decisions today about what we should and should not do to minimize our chance of developing cancer, it makes sense to play down the hypothetical and emphasize the known.

Third, some of the known cancer "high risk factors" pose more of a health hazard than do others. Similarly, some of the eight categories of cancer-causing factors discussed here are more within our control than are others.

Fourth, we do not have to have "all the answers" about a known high-risk factor before making a recommendation on how to reduce one's chances of developing cancer. If a chemical or lifestyle has been shown, in a multitude of human studies, to increase the frequency of cancer, we need not await an explanation of *how* it causes cancer before deciding to act on the information.

In addition to identifying the known cancer high-risk factors around us, the chapters which follow will look closely at what types of evidence have been accumulated and *how* scientists reached their conclusions about cancer causation. The research we're dealing with here did not revolve around cases of white-coated professors, emerging from their laboratory shrieking, "Eureka!" and an-

nouncing that they had the ultimate answer to the cancer mystery.
Research and discovery about human cancer causation has, at least
so far, been a slow, step by step process, much more oriented
toward the study of people than to chemicals in test tubes or
animals in laboratory cages.

In some of the cases you'll read about, the identification of the
human carcinogen occurred relatively dramatically, the result of
the astute observations of "medical detectives" who noted an unusual number of illnesses or deaths from specific causes among
particular groups of individuals. For instance, those working in the
same occupational setting, those exposed to the same drug. In at
least one instance (the investigation of tobacco as a possible cancer-
causing agent), the initial discoveries were rendered less dramatic
by the failure of those who were personally or professionally com-
mitted to the use of cigarettes to accept the obvious fact that smoking increased manyfold one's odds of developing cancer of many
sites. This resistance necessitated repeated searches for "more
proof," and this diluted the effect of what under other conditions
would have been a startling announcement with profound implications for a large segment of our population.

But in still other cases, implication of a chemical or behavior pattern as a "high-risk" factor in cancer, occurred more subtly, gradually over the years as a result of the efforts of scientists from many
disciplines all over the world. For example, the role of excessive
sun exposure in causing skin cancer was not defined in any one day
or year. Evidence simply accumulated over the course of six or
seven decades.

The differences in the manner in which scientists identified
cancer risk factors influenced the lengths and writing style of the
various chapters of this book. Some chapters will assume the characteristics of a medical mystery story, introducing actual case histories and the medical detectives who unfolded the "whodunnit" of
that type of cancer. In these instances, only the names of the victims will be changed. Other chapters will reflect the fact that the
"discovery" occurred over a period of years, without any particular
fanfare.

In all chapters, I have attempted to minimize statistics, tables, graphs, and other excess scientific baggage in order to keep the text as readable as possible.

Preventing Cancer is an optimistic book on a depressing subject. It is an attempt to make a frightening disease less frightening by putting the floodlights on it. Cancer should not be a disease which is lurking in the shadows. It is not an inevitable result of being human. The more we learn about malignancies and their origins, the more we realize that much of our fate is in our own hands.

ELIZABETH WHELAN

New York City

ACKNOWLEDGMENTS

A significant number of individuals offered their time and expertise to the preparation of this book. I extend particular thanks to members of the National Cancer Institute, including Dr. W. Gary Flamm, Assistant Director of the Division of Cancer Cause and Prevention; Dr. Marvin A. Schneiderman, Associate Director for Field Studies and Statistics; Division of Cancer Cause and Prevention; Dr. Joseph F. Fraumeni, and Dr. Robert Hoover of the Environmental Epidemiology Branch, and the many representatives of the American Cancer Institute, including Dr. E. Cuyler Hammond, Vice President (Epidemiology and Statistics); Dr. G. Congdon Wood, Director of the Society's Section on Unproven Methods of Cancer Management; and Edwin Silverberg, Project Statistician.

Additionally, I benefited from the comments of Dr. Fredrick J. Stare, Professor of Nutrition at the Harvard School of Public Health; Dr. Philip Cole, Associate Professor of Epidemiology, Harvard School of Public Health; Dr. Ernst L. Wynder (President), Dr. Bandaru S. Reddy, Penny Ashwanden, and Angelica T. Cantlon, American Health Foundation; Dr. John Zapp and Leavitt S. White, E. I. du Pont de Nemours and Company; Robert B. Downey and Dr. Maurice Johnson, B. F. Goodrich; Dr. Richard W. McBurney, Diamond Shamrock Corporation; Dr. Vernon Riley, Pacific Northwest Research Foundation in Seattle; Dr. Albert C. Kolbye, Associate Director for Sciences, Bureau of Foods, Food and Drug Administration; Dr. David Schottenfeld, Director of Epidemiology, Memorial Sloan Kettering Cancer Center; Dr. William Nicholson, Mount Sinai Environmental Sciences Department; Dr. Farrington Daniels, Jr., Professor of Medicine and Head of the Dermatology Division,

New York Hospital-Cornell Medical Center; Dr. Charles Black, Executive Vice President, Council for Agricultural Science and Technology; Dr. Thomas H. Jukes, Professor of Medical Physics, University of California at Berkeley; Dr. Judith Goldberg, Mount Sinai School of Medicine; Dr. Paula H. Kanarek, Assistant Professor of Statistics, Oregon State University at Corvallis; Dr. Perry Robins, Associate Professor of Clinical Dermatology, New York University Medical Center; Dr. William D. Bloomer, Assistant Professor, of Radiation Therapy, Harvard Medical School; Jerome Heckman, Dr. Daniel S. Dixler, Dr. Wilhelm C. Hueper, and Robert Ferrante.

This work is based on the analysis of several hundred medical and scientific documents, but three publications were especially useful in my research: *Persons at High Risk of Cancer: An Approach to Cancer Etiology and Control,* edited by Dr. Joseph F. Fraumeni, published by the Academic Press; *Cancer Epidemiology and Prevention,* edited by Dr. David Schottenfeld, published by Charles C. Thomas; and the proceedings of the Symposium on Nutrition in the Causation of Cancer, published in the November 1975 issue of *Cancer Research.* Additionally, the papers and discussions presented at the "Origins of Human Cancer" meeting (September 7–September 14, 1976) arranged jointly by the Cold Spring Harbor Laboratory and the Harvard School of Public Health, proved invaluable in providing a background on the etiology of cancer.

Finally, I would like to express my thanks to June Miller who typed the many drafts of this manuscript, to my husband Stephen T. Whelan who took the time to read and appraise each version, and to the New York Academy of Medicine and New York Public Libraries for their courteous and efficient assistance in locating the vast quantity of research material which was vital to the preparation of this book.

Preventing Cancer

1

WHAT CAUSES HUMAN CANCER?

> "Happy he who could learn the causes of things and who put beneath his feet all fears."
>
> Virgil, Georgics I, Line 490

Cancer, derived from the Greek word for crab, *karkinos,* stands for a large, varied group of diseases, capable of afflicting plants, animals, and man, which can arise in any organ or tissue. The main characteristic of cancer is abnormal, undisciplined, seemingly unrestricted, growth of body cells, with the resultant masses compressing, invading, and destroying contiguous tissue. If not caught and controlled in an early stage, these cells are capable of setting up secondary colonies (that is, of metastasizing) and causing further invasion of tissue.

BIOLOGY OR ENVIRONMENT?

Until relatively recently, much of the focus in cancer causation research was on genetic and family susceptibility. The view was that those of us who eventually do develop cancer were genetically programmed to do so. It was thus considered part of God's will, out of our control. With this interpretation of causation, it is no wonder that cancer has traditionally been spoken of in whispers and people who "had it in the family" felt defeated from the start of life.

Some individuals are at high risk of cancer because of their chromosome structure and will develop the disease apparently without outside cause. For example, those with Down's syndrome (mongolism) have eleven times or more the normal risk of developing acute leukemia. But Down's syndrome and the very few other genetic conditions which directly predispose individuals to cancer are extremely rare and here, in our personal quest to avoid cancer, are not worthy of practical consideration.[1]

Of somewhat greater interest is the concept of family susceptibility. The aggregation of cancer in families is a well-documented phenomenon dating back to the seventeenth century. Individuals whose mother, father, or siblings develop cancer of the stomach, breast, large intestine, uterus, or lung have a two- to fourfold greater chance of themselves developing the specific form of cancer. If one twin develops the disease, the other runs a greater chance than a nonrelated individual of following the same pattern. Brain tumors and sarcomas seem to occur more frequently than expected in brothers and sisters of children with these tumors.

The limited data available do suggest some increased familial risk of developing cancer of the same site for certain forms of the disease. But the question here is: Is the "family susceptibility" due to some genetic patterns or were the family members exposed to the same type of external environment, following the same lifestyles and, as a result, developing the same disease?

The family susceptibility arguments versus the environmentally induced ones are much like the chicken and egg question. One might argue that a red-haired, blue-eyed, fair-skinned woman whose mother developed skin cancer is "destined" to develop this disease. But, on the other hand, she probably will not be affected

---

1. There is another type of disease disposition to cancer. For instance, patients with ulcerative colitis and pernicious anemia are routinely considered to be at high risk of colon and stomach cancer respectively. Attention to these risks are standard in medical practice.

unless she exposes her skin to an excessive amount of sunlight. So which factor is more important? Family susceptibility or environment? In terms of prevention, the fact that she has some control over the sun exposure factor, but not over her family history, makes the environmental aspect more important.

If you have a family history of some form of cancer, particularly when that form of cancer afflicted your relative at an early age, say prior to sixty, there are two practical ways you can use that information.

First, inform your personal physician of this fact. Second, be particularly aware of the factors within your control which might further increase your risk of that disease. For instance, individuals who smoke a pack of cigarettes each day but do not have a family history of cancer of the lung, will run a four- to sixfold greater risk of developing this disease as compared to those who do not smoke and have no family history of this carcinoma. But one-pack-a-day smokers whose parents or other first-degree relatives have lung cancer run a fifteenfold increased risk of developing carcinoma of the lung.

Research on genetic susceptibility to various types of cancer is still a very active field. And results could have some very practical applications: for instance, if we knew exactly why some people who smoke develop lung cancer, while some others do not, we might be able to tell one smoker, "Hey buddy, you're the one. You've got the genetic code with the potential for cancer of the lung," and tell another he was not in the high-risk cancer group (of course, this smoker would still be facing increased risks from heart disease, emphysema, and other cigarette-related afflictions). Presumably if you knew you were sure to get lung cancer, you wouldn't smoke.

But despite the continuing interest in the role of a possible biological predisposition in cancer development, research on cancer causes over the past thirty years has confirmed that external factors far override any internal ones. Indeed it is now widely accepted that 70 to 90 percent of all human cancer is induced by environmental causes. "Environmental" here is used in a very broad sense, encompassing personal habits, life-styles, as well as "chemicals" around us.

This is good news. It means that, once we identify the causes, cancer will be, at least to some extent, within our control. The relatively new emphasis on the environment is based in a large part on international studies. As will be discussed in this chapter, the facts that there is such a wide variation in cancer death rates around the world, and people who migrate from their native land assume the disease characteristics of their new country, suggests that external influences, not biology, are responsible.

CANCER AND THE CONCEPT OF "CAUSE"

In London in 1849, John Snow noticed that there was a sudden increase in the number of cases of cholera. After some detective work, he concluded that the victims were not evenly distributed around the city, but rather all lived in one geographic area. Once he made that observation it did not take him long to implicate the sewage-contaminated water which was flowing from the infamous Broad Street Pump.

Snow had isolated the "cause" of the cholera epidemic: contaminated water. Of course, the actual cause was the cholera microorganism. But for practical purposes, it was the polluted water that was making people sick.

Establishing cancer causation and deciding what to do about it is not that simple. There are three basic ways in which the study of a chronic disease like cancer is different from that of a communicable disease like cholera.

The Time Difference

In communicable disease, it is a matter of a few days or a few weeks between the time the victim is exposed and the time he develops the disease. Not so with cancer. It can easily be ten, twenty, thirty years or more between the time we are exposed, or begin to expose ourselves to the cause, and the time we notice symptoms. This makes the study of cancer causation very difficult. When Dr. Snow went to the scene to investigate the cholera epidemic, the same people were there as were there the week before. The pump was still there. Circumstances hadn't changed. But when a cancer epidemiologist, that is, a medical investigator interested in the causes of cancer, begins to search for leads, the cancer equivalent of the pump may be gone, the victims dispersed or perhaps dead from other causes.

In 1849, not everyone who drank from the Broad Street pump developed cholera, nor were all existing cholera cases explained by exposure to water from the pump. But the evidence was immediately at hand and convincing enough that the cause was accepted. There was no need for elaborate statistical exercises to prove the relationship between the contamination and the illness. But because of the difference in the amount of time elapsed between exposure and onset of symptoms of disease, the nature of the proof for cancer causation must be stronger. As with the cholera situation, not 100 percent of people exposed to a known cancer-promoting factor will develop the disease. Perhaps they were not exposed long enough, had some special immunity, or died of heart disease or something else before cancer was diagnosed. Whatever the reason, *the long latency period of cancer necessitates that the concept of cause be based on statistical association.* Cause here means that in the absence of exposure to the factor, the disease in question would have occurred less frequently.

There are still those who want to brush off recent discoveries in the area of human cancer causation by noting that "statistics are just a group of numbers looking for an argument" and that "statisticians are people who collect data and draw confusions." But the fact remains that in making a cause-effect link for the many forms of cancer, statistical associations are the primary means.

If the disease we're talking about is a rare form of liver carcinoma and shows up in one group of workers in a chemical industry, the statistical association is a relatively uncomplicated one. But if the disease is a common one—like lung cancer—and affecting different people from different walks of life, the statistical association must be based on thousands of individuals who are exposed to the suspected cause, and thousands who are not exposed to the suspected cause. To confirm the association, that is, that the factor is a cause of the disease, further questions must be asked:

—*Are people who are exposed to greater amounts of the suspected factor more likely to get the disease than are those who are exposed to less of it?* In other words, is there a dose-response relationship? Are heavy smokers more likely to develop lung cancer than light smokers?

—*Do all or most studies show the same results?*

—*Do the results make sense in terms of time trends?* For instance, is the hypothesis that cigarettes cause cancer consistent with what we know about which types of cancer are rising?

—*What happens when you remove the suspected factor?* Do people who stop smoking diminish their odds of developing cancer?

—*Do populations who, because of their lifestyle are not exposed to the factor, develop the disease less frequently?* Do Mormons and Seventh Day Adventists whose religion prohibits cigarette smoking have lower rates of lung cancer?

In epidemiologically establishing a cause of cancer, the goal is to confirm the consistency of the observations.

A *Multitude of Factors*

Unlike in the classification of cholera, different scientists have different definitions of what is and what is not cancer. Some might limit their definition to the presence of a malignant tumor. Others may feel that a benign tumor is in some instances the first step of what will eventually be a malignant process.

Even more important, unlike the case of infectious disease, some cancer-causing agents may need the presence of other chemicals before they become active. Animal experiments at least suggest that this is a possibility for humans. For instance, when the known animal carcinogen bracken fern, a natural plant that looks much like an asparagus and is used in some parts of the world as a food for humans, is fed to rats, very few of them develop bladder tumors. But if these animals are given an extra dose of the vitamin thiamine, over half of them develop bladder tumors. On the other hand, vitamin A, when fed with a known cancer-causing agent, has been shown to inhibit various types of cancers in laboratory animals.

The cause-effect pattern in cancer is not always on a 1:1 basis. This multifaceted aspect of the cancer-causation puzzle helps explain why not everyone who is exposed to a carcinogen develops the disease. Again, the critical factor in the study of cancer causation is the observation of increased risk.

What to Do about It

When Snow made his association between the pump and cholera, the problem was clear and the necessary action was obvious: close off the pump, eliminate the cause of the disease.

When it comes to a cause or possible cause of cancer, it is not that easy. As we'll see in later chapters, it is sometimes absolutely impossible to eliminate carcinogens, even when they have been shown to cause cancer in humans. In excess amounts, exposure to the sun causes skin cancer. Obviously, we are neither going to ban the sun or issue an edict that everyone with blond hair and blue eyes must stay indoors in the daytime. We must learn to live with this potential risk, adapt our behavior so we can coexist with it in relative safety.

Similarly, certain forms of medical treatment—X rays, for instance—have been shown in some specific circumstances to increase the risk of human cancer. But X rays are an essential diagnostic tool. We must learn to use them safely. Certain industrial chemicals, for instance vinyl chloride used in the production of plastics, have been linked with a rare form of human liver cancer. But, again, a general banning of all plastic products is not the answer.

There are three key concepts which have emerged to distinguish the acute diseases which afflicted our grandparents from the chronic ones which threaten us today. First, the need to quantify risk, acknowledging that there is a difference between a high dose which may indeed present a hazard to man's health and a low dose which will have no effect at all. Second, the necessity of weighing the benefits of a given substance versus its possible risks. Third, the reality that there is no such thing as "proving something safe". In studying substances, we are by definition looking for harmful effects. Anything could eventually be proven to be harmful. We can only make intelligent decision after rationally examining the information we have. The concept of safety is a relative one.

MEDICAL DETECTION

What do you think of when you hear the term "cancer research"? Very likely you picture a medical laboratory full of white-coated scientists, test tubes, and caged experimental animals. You may well think that it is this group of individuals who are, alone, working toward an understanding of the causes of human cancer.

Actually, however, the most fruitful forms of cancer research over the past two centuries have not been performed by scientists in laboratories. Indeed most of our current awareness of all known causes of human cancer is the direct result of the detective work of epidemiologists,[2] those medical scientists who analyze groups or clusters of individuals who manifest high or low incidences of disease, in this case a form of cancer.

Scientists have now identified eight categories of circumstances which place human beings at high risk of cancer. In all eight instances described in this book, the classification "human cancer risk" was applied only after a number—in some cases hundreds of thousands—of human beings died following exposure to that chemical or physical agent. The nature of cancer epidemiology is that we are learning from the tragic experiences of others. The goal of this pursuit is, obviously, to institute measures that will prevent the recurrence of the same tragedies.

The Clues

In looking for factors which increase risks of cancer, the epidemiologist has a number of tools. One obvious one is to look at the

2. An epidemiologist is a medical scientist who studies the cause and distribution of disease in a population. *Epidemiology* is a word invented by Hippocrates four hundred years before the Christian era.

worldwide geographic distribution of cancer. As we'll illustrate in a later chapter, there are significant differences from country to country in general cancer death rates and those of selected site. For instance, the stomach cancer rate in Japan is five times higher than that in the United States. On the other hand, Japanese women have a remarkably lower death rate from breast cancer than do women from the United States, Canada, England and Wales, and Switzerland. Liver cancer deaths occur very frequently in many African countries, very infrequently in North America and Europe. Cancer of the cervix is a rare disease in Israel, a common one in Colombia, South America, Puerto Rico, and among non-white women in the United States.

These are epidemiological clues, leads which suggest that something peculiar to those countries or groups is responsible for their relatively high rates of specific forms of cancer.

But, you say, perhaps it is really a genetic difference between persons of different nationalities. Perhaps the breast cancer rate is low and stomach cancer death rate high in Japan because Japanese people have a peculiar resistance and susceptibility respectively to these two diseases. That would be possible, except that an additional epidemiological clue makes it highly unlikely: when Japanese men and women move to the United States, live here for a generation or more and presumably assimilate various aspects of our culture, their breast cancer and stomach cancer rates become similar to those of native Americans. The conclusion is that something in the Japanese lifestyle accounts for their unique cancer pattern.

The study of geographic disease patterns has recently been applied to the United States as a whole. And interesting results have emerged. Certain counties in Minnesota, northern Michigan, Wisconsin, and the Dakotas, have an unusually high mortality rate of stomach cancer for both sexes. This suggests that there is something to which both men and women are exposed, perhaps an unusual diet of a particular ethnic group, which is to blame. In some counties of New Jersey there is excess mortality from bladder cancer—but only among men. The fact that the excessive mortality is limited to men suggests that some occupational factor is involved.

This type of "clustering" is the most significant tool the epidemiologist has. And it is obviously not limited to the study of geographic areas. It was the unusual clustering of lung cancer among smokers, of breast cancer among nuns, of leukemia among radiologists, of skin cancer among outdoor laborers, of liver cancer among a small group of vinyl chloride workers which led to the description of the causes of these diseases.

The Limitations and Advantages

Epidemiology and the study of the clustering of human cancer has not yet provided all the answers. A primary limitation of epidemiological analysis of cancer causation is that it is an "after the fact" process. It does not offer us the possibility of predicting whether a substance *will* increase cancer risk. Additionally, the epidemiological method is more useful in detecting a rare disease that is caused by one type of exposure than it is in explaining causation of a widespread disease which may be the result of many different types of risk. For instance when a rare disease like mesothelioma (cancer of the lining of the chest or abdominal cavity, a disease which so far has been invariably fatal) was observed to occur with unusual frequency among asbestos workers, the study to establish cause could proceed in a straightforward manner. But with a common disease like breast cancer which may be related to more than one risk factor, the epidemiological quest for causation is more difficult.

On the other hand, from our point of view in attempting to minimize our risks of developing cancer, the information on cancer causation developed from epidemiological studies is the most convincing evidence we have. It involves real people, real-life circumstances. And in each of the eight chapters on "known high-risk factors," the epidemiological evidence is convincing enough to warrant our attention.

CAN'T WE PREDICT THAT SOMETHING WILL CAUSE CANCER IN HUMANS?

Do people have to die in order for us to acknowledge that a substance is harmful? Can't we test things to make sure they are safe before we expose ourselves to them?

We don't hear very much about the successes in the field of cancer prevention. Only the failures get the headlines. But the fact is that through animal testing, scientists have been able to identify chemicals which seem to have a significant potential for causing human cancer. These chemicals are kept out of our food, water, drugs, and workplace. No rational person would want to have human beings exposed to moderate or high levels of a chemical which at low doses caused malignant tumors in different types of animals. Thousands of chemicals are now kept out of our environment or are carefully regulated because they are powerful animal carcinogens. Scientists *are* taking preventive measures.

But the identification of a potential human cancer-causing agent is a difficult and controversial area. The questions boil down to: How many different animal experiments do you have to do before you conclude that it is not safe for humans to come in contact with it? If massive doses of the chemical cause some cancers in some animals, should that mean that humans should never be allowed to come in contact with even minute traces of it, even though the substance is invaluable, perhaps lifesaving, in some circumstances?

A very small number of scientists feel that once a chemical has been shown to cause cancer in any animal in any circumstances it should be immediately suspected of causing cancer in man too and, in the interest of safety, should be banned. Initially, this might sound reasonable. After all, who would want to take a chance? Why not err on the side of caution rather than run the risk of new tragedies?

If there were two neat categories, 1) "cancer-causing agents" which we can live without; and 2) "non-cancer-causing agents" which we need, that type of philosophy would be appropriate. But this is not the situation. Some useful, indeed, vital, chemicals, for instance vitamin A, penicillin, isoniazid (considered a "miracle drug" in the control of tuberculosis), phenobarbital cause an increased risk of cancer in some animals, although not all, yet are presumably safe in appropriate doses for human use.

Some chemicals cause cancer in animals in very high doses but not in moderate or low doses. And some chemicals which are carcinogenic in animals but pose no known risk to us in the manner in which they are used, are necessary to protect human health and maintain our high standard of living.

We can continue to use animal experiments to predict risks for human beings, but we must do so using scientific judgment and a hefty amount of common sense.

2

A CANCER EPIDEMIC?

"The news tonight is that the United States is number one in cancer. The National Cancer Institute estimates that if you're living in America your chances of getting cancer are higher than anywhere else in the world."

> Dan Rather
> CBS Reports Special
> The American Way of Cancer
> October 15, 1975

"It's now known that increased contamination of our air, water and food is contributing to our *soaring* cancer rates. . . . " [Italics mine]

> Leslie Stahl
> CBS Reports Special
> The Politics of Cancer
> June 22, 1976

If present trends continue, one in four Americans alive today, over fifty-four million people, will eventually develop cancer. Over the years, some form of cancer will strike two out of every three families. In 1977, over 385,000 Americans died of cancer, a rate of about one every one and a half minutes, 1,055 people a day.

The figures are both staggering and understandably frightening. But before we can begin any discussion about what we can do to diminish our risk, we must put those statistics and their implications in sharper focus.

As recently as ten years ago, *cancer* was not a word that appeared very frequently in the headlines. It was hardly ever the subject of an hour-long television show or a topic covered in depth in a woman's magazine. Now the topic commands a significant amount of attention; "DES, a Cancer Causing Agent in Meat"; "Aldrin and Dieldrin, Pesticides Suspected of Causing Cancer, Banned"; "Cancer Hazard in Plastic Wrap"; "Cancer Hazard in Plastic Soft-Drink Bottles"; "Children's Sleepwear Treated with Cancer-Causing TRIS"; "Critics Say Carcinogens Used To Decaffeinate Coffee"; "Red Dye Number 2 Causes Tumors in Laboratory Animals"; "Saccharin, Suspected Cancer Agent, May Be Banned."

The television reports on cancer pick up where the headlines leave off. A few years ago, for example, CBS Special Reports, "The American Way of Cancer" and "The Politics of Cancer," showed scenes of polluted streams and city air, contaminated workplaces, chemists peering into suspicious-looking test tubes, fields being sprayed with insecticides and food labels with a string of unpronounceable polysyllabic names, and the message both specifically, as the above quotes document, and implicitly, was that we were in the grip of a cancer epidemic, one which was having a particularly devasting effect on industrialized countries like the United States.

No wonder people think the U.S. is "number one" in cancer, now experiencing "soaring rates."

Cancer Trends

The cancer picture in this country is depressing enough already without exaggerating the situation with misinformation. So here let's set the record straight.

First, assertions of the media notwithstanding, our cancer death rate is not "soaring." According to 1977 *Cancer Facts and Figures* published by the American Cancer Society, *the overall incidence of cancer has decreased slightly since 1950.* The age adjusted death rate from malignancies has increased, from about 125 cancer deaths per 100,000 population in 1950, to about 131 per 100,000 in 1975, but this is by no means dramatic enough to warrant the words "epidemic" or "soaring."

It is true that cancer deaths were relatively less common during the first decade of this century. But it's essential to take into account that the life expectancy of the average man and woman was rather limited back then. For instance, a white male child born between 1900 and 1903 could, at the time of birth, expect to live only forty-eight years. Today the life expectancy for males at birth is over seventy years. Men and women born in the early part of the century generally died of scarlet fever, whooping cough, diphtheria, pneumonia, influenza, or tuberculosis before cancer had a chance to affect them.

In 1975 the press reported a sudden, and what they considered startling, shift in the cancer death rate in this country, specifically, a reported 5.2 percent increase in cancer mortality during the first seven months of 1975. There was much speculation about an environmental "cancer time bomb" going off and the National Cancer Institute received hundreds of telephone calls a day during the height of the scare, requesting information which would explain the apparent epidemic of cancer. This incident demonstrated some of the severe problems with using preliminary disease statistics to make judgments. It was later found that instead of a 5.2 percent increase, there had been a 0.7 percent (age-adjusted) increase in the cancer death rate, the discrepancy explained in part by the fact that the preliminary figures were not age-adjusted or representative of trends in the country as a whole.

Second, in developing your own personal cancer plan, one set of "facts and figures" should be of interest to you. As an American, you are not at equal risk of developing all types of cancer. Some forms of the disease are more likely to affect you than others.

As you read about the known risks of human cancer, keep in mind these priorities. The preventive measures which will minimize your odds on these four forms of cancer deserve your most intense attention.

The Three Leading Causes of Cancer Death in the United States[a]

	MALE	FEMALE
#1	lung	breast
	(68,300)	(33,700)
#2	colon & rectum	colon & rectum
	(24,800)	(26,500)
#3	prostate gland	lung
	(20,100)	(20,700)

[a] and the estimated number of Americans who died from them in 1977.

SOURCE: *1977 Cancer Facts and Figures,* American Cancer Society

Third, although there has been a slight rise in cancer mortality in the past thirty years, not all forms of cancer death have increased. Some (like cancer of the breast, colon-rectum) have remained about the same, and others (for instance, cancer of the stomach) have declined precipitously.

On the other hand, lung cancer, the number one cause of cancer death in men, has increased by more than *twenty-five times* in the past forty-five years. And the death rate is going up steadily for women. Smaller increases in death rates and/or incidence have been noted for cancer of the pancreas, prostate, ovary, and male bladder.

But, as the proverb goes, "Words are but wind, but seeing is believing." So selected cancer statistics are graphically presented below:[1]

Chart I shows the total number of deaths per year caused by cancer. The trend is obvious: the number of deaths from this cause in the United States has been increasing. But, on the other hand, the graph is misleading as it does not take into account the fact that the population has increased almost threefold since 1900.

1. This sequence of charts on cancer trends originally appeared in a paper entitled "Cancer: A Statement of the Facts" by T. H. Cox of E. I. du Pont de Nemours and Company, 1976, and is used with permission.

CHART I

Number of Cancer Deaths in the United States

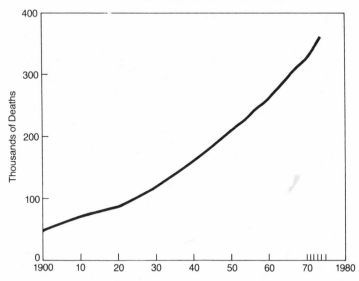

SOURCE: 1900–1940 Calculated from population, *Statistical Abstract of the United States 1970,* Table No. 2, p. 5, U.S. Bureau of Census, 91st edition; and from death rates, *Vital Statistics of the United States, 1950* Vol I, Table 8.30, National Office of Vital Statistics, 1954.

1950–1969 *Mortality Trends for Leading Causes of Death, United States 1950–1969,* Table 3, Department of Health, Education and Welfare, Pub. No. (HRA) 74-1853, 1974.

1972 *General Mortality 1972* Volume II, Section 1, Table 1-13.

1974 *Monthly Vital Statistics Report - Advance Report Final Mortality Statistics, 1974,* p. 11, National Center for Health Statistics, February 3, 1976.

Chart II shows the number of cancer deaths in the U.S. per 100,000 population, that is, taking into account changes in the total population in the U.S. But without an age adjustment, the trend is still somewhat misleading.

CHART II

Cancer Death Rates in the United States

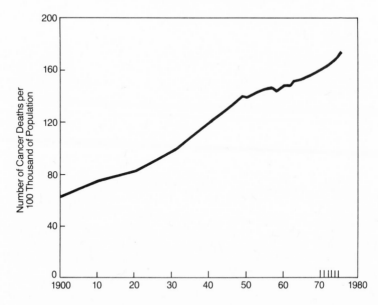

SOURCE: 1900–1950 *Vital Statistics of the United States, 1950* Vol. I, Table 8.30,
National Office of Vital Statistics, 1954.

1950–1969 *Mortality Trends for Leading Causes of Death, United
States 1950–1969,* Table 2, Department of Health, Education and Welfare Pub. No. (HRA) 74-1853, 1974.

1970–1972 *General Mortality Tables 1972,* Vol. II, Section 1, Table
1-7.

1974 *Monthly Vital Statistics Report—Advance Report Final Mortality
Statistics, 1974,* p. 11, National Center for Health Statistics, February 3,
1976.

1975 *Monthly Vital Statistics Report—Provisional Statistics,* p. 7, National Center for Health Statistics, March 31, 1976.

Chart III shows the cancer death rate in the United States per 100,000
population adjusted for age, that is, taking into account the fact that the
population is older in recent years (and thus more cancer prone) than it
was, for example, in the 1940's and 1950's. Obviously, the upward trend in
cancer death rates is not as marked when you take age changes into account.

CHART III

Cancer Death Rates in the United States

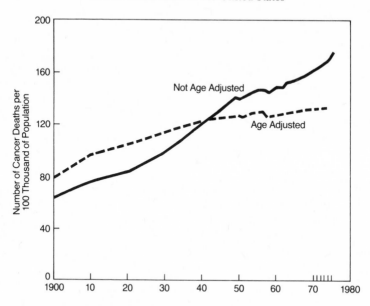

SOURCE: Age-adjusted cancer death rates:
     1900–1940 Age-specific death rates from *Vital Statistics of the United States, 1950,* Vol. I, Table 8.30 and Table 2.21, National Office of Vital Statistics, 1954, for 1940 population.
     1950–1969 *Mortality Trends for Leading Causes of Death, United States 1950–1969,* Table C, Department of Health, Education and Welfare Pub. No. (HRA) 74-1853, 1974.
     1974 Age-specific death rates from *Monthly Vital Statistics Report— Advance Report Final Mortality Statistics, 1974,* pp. 14 and 15, National Center for Health Statistics, February 3, 1976.

The next step in analyzing the data on cancer trends is to recognize, first, that cancer death rates for men and women are different, and second, that there are differences in death rates due to cancer in various organs of the body. Chart IV is particularly revealing, indicating that contrary to popular belief *there is no general cancer epidemic in this country. The epidemic is limited to lung cancer.*

CHART IV

Age-Adjusted Cancer Death Rates in the United States for Men

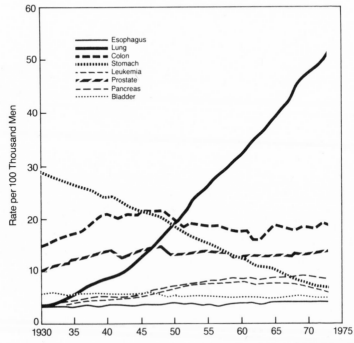

SOURCE: *Ca: A Cancer Journal for Clinicians,* pp. 18 and 19. Published by the American Cancer Society, Jan.–Feb. 1976.

Chart V shows that the total cancer death rate in the United States for men is increasing, but if cancer of the respiratory system, overwhelmingly the result of cigarette smoking, is eliminated, *then the overall cancer death rate for men would be decreasing.*

CHART V

Age-Adjusted Total Cancer Death Rates in the United States for Men

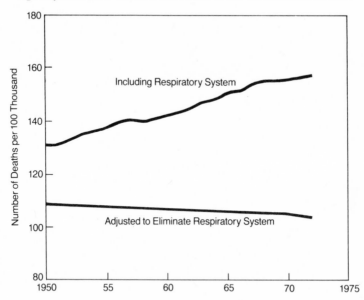

SOURCE: Mortality Trends for Leading Causes of Death, United States, 1950–1969, Table C, Department of Health, Education and Welfare, Pub. No. (HRA) 74-1853.

1950 *Vital Statistics of the United States*, 1950, Vol. I, Table 8.43, pp. 210 and 211.

1960 *Vital Statistics of the United States*, 1960, Vol. II, Mortality, Part A. Table 1-M, p. 1-27.

1970 *Vital Statistics of the United States*, 1970, Vol. II, Mortality, Part A, Table 1-19, pp. 1-9 and 1-10.

1972 *Vital Statistics for the United States*, 1972, Vol. II, Table 1-8, pp. 1-10 and 1-11.

The adjustment to eliminate respiratory cancer was made by subtracting the age-specific death rates for respiratory cancer from the age-specific total death rate and then multiplying by the 1940 population.

Chart VI displays trends in mortality rates in eight important sites of cancer in women in the U.S. Deaths due to cancer of the stomach and uterus are decreasing. Deaths due to cancers at other sites do not show any dramatic increases except lung cancer. Lung cancer for women has begun to increase recently due to an increase in cigarette smoking by women which began in the 1940s.

CHART VI

Age-Adjusted Cancer Death Rates in the United States For Women

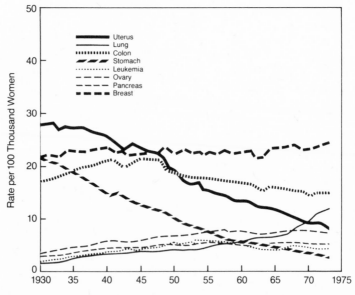

SOURCE: *Ca: A Cancer Journal for Clinicians,* pp. 18 and 19. Published by the American Cancer Society, Jan.–Feb. 1976.

Selected Cancer Death Rates (All Sites)
Around the World[a]

	MALE	FEMALE
Luxembourg	212	115
Austria	192	126
England and Wales	185	119
Switzerland	172	109
United States	156	107
Canada	154	108
Japan	140	91
Thailand	25	17

[a] Age adjusted death rates per 100,000 population for selected countries.
SOURCE: *World Health Statistics Annual,* 1970–1971.

Again, and it's worth repeating, as is evident from the chart sequence, if it were not for the sudden and continuing upswing in the lung-cancer death rate starting in 1930, the general American death rate from cancer would have been stabilizing or declining.

Fourth, the United States is not "number one in cancer" as is so often alleged. There is significant variation from country to country in the general mortality from cancer and, as we'll comment on later, by particular cancer site. The range is from 212 male cancer deaths per 100,000 in Luxembourg, to 25 per 100,000 in Thailand. The United States falls in between with a cancer death rate for men of 156.

Thus, as you can tell from this brief overview of statistics and trends, the cancer picture in the United States is neither frightfully grim nor totally depressing. And there are, as will be detailed in the next eight chapters, some measures you can take to protect yourself from some of the most frequently occurring forms of this disease.

PART I

Factors Known
to Increase Your Odds
on Developing Cancer

3

TOBACCO

"Cigarettes are killers that travel in packs."
Mary S. Ott

TOBACCO: CONDEMNATION AND PRAISE

"A custome loathsome to the eye, hatefull to the Nose, harmeful to
the braine, dangerous to the Lungs, and in the blacke stinking
fume thereof neerest resembling the horrible Stigian smoke of the
pit that is bottemlesse . . . for it is a stinking loathsome thing and
so is hell. . . . If I were to invite the devil to dinner, he should
have three dishes: first a pig; second a pull and ling of mustard and
a pipe of tobacco."

With those words in 1604, King James I of Great Britain condemned the use of tobacco. He wished that Sir Walter Raleigh and
Sir Francis Drake had never introduced England to the habit in
the 1580s. He probably regretted that Columbus was so fascinated
when he saw the natives of San Salvador blowing clouds of smoke
from their nostrils that he brought some back with him and started
a chain of events which led to tobacco use in Spain, France, England, and all over Europe.

Tobacco has been a source of controversy among physicians and
laymen for hundreds of years. While King James and others were
condemning it, placing heavy taxes on its sale, and threatening
penalties which included nose amputation, others were proclaim-

ing its magical medical potential. "Herba Panacea" was at some point recommended to cure cancer, epilepsy, arthritis and "other diseases of the Lunges and Inward Partes." Real enthusiasts whose love for tobacco was obviously blind claimed "it maketh the voice clear . . . it maketh the breath sweet."

The generalized health warnings and predictions of loss of morality attributed to tobacco had little effect on its growing popularity for use in pipes, snuffing, and chewing. And although for each advocate of tobacco use there was an equally vociferous nonuser who condemned it, in the first 250 years after the tobacco plant was brought from the new world, there were no verified and circulated reports that tobacco was linked with cancer. There were, of course, clinical opinions expressed to the effect that tobacco was harmful to physical well-being. For instance in the late seventeenth century, a Dr. Evard of London wrote that "tobacco causes vomit and is an enemy of the stomach." But cancer wasn't mentioned as a by-product of smoking any more than was any other disease.

It was in 1761 that an English physician made the first clinical report documenting that tobacco use causes cancer. In that year Dr. John Hill presented his *Cautions Against the Immoderate Use of Snuff.* He reported two cases of cancer of the nose, both victims having "polypusses" which he believed to be malignant. He described the first case in his historically significant document:

> This unfortunate gentleman, after a long and immoderate use of Snuff, perceived that he breathed with difficulty through one of his nostrils; the complaint gradually encreased, 'til he perceived a swelling within. . . . It grew slowly, 'til, in the end, it filled up that whole nostril, and swelled the nose so as to obstruct the breathing . . . he found it necessary to then apply for assistance. The swelling was quite black and it adhered by a broad base, so that it was impossible to attempt the getting it away . . . and the consequence was a discharge of a thin sharp humour with dreadful pain, and all the frightful symptoms of cancer . . . and he seemed without hope when I last saw him.

His second case was also a victim of the snuff:

> The person was a lady of a sober and virtuous life . . . she had long been accustomed to Snuff and took it in a very great quantity . . . she

felt a strange soreness in the upper part of her nostril . . . after a little time, came on a discharge of a very offensive matter; not in any quantity but of an intolerable smell, and was more so to her, as she was naturally a person of great delicacy. The discharge encreased, and it soon became necessary for her to leave off Snuff. A surgeon was employed, but to very little purpose. . . .

Dr. Hill in 1761 was describing malignancies. And he placed the blame squarely on tobacco, in the form of snuff, which according to modern evidence probably did cause the lesions.

His observations, however, were not the type that would merit headlines. People kept smoking, chewing, and sniffing.

Through the 1800s there were some random reports suggesting that cancer and tobacco use were linked. (Until late in this century tobacco use meant pipes, cigars, chewing tobacco, and snuff. No one ever heard of a cigarette.) A Boston surgeon in 1849 wrote that "for more than twenty years back I have been in the habit of inquiring of patients who come to me with cancers . . . of the gums, tongue and lips . . . whether they use tobacco. . . . When, as is usually the case, one side of the tongue is affected with ulcerated cancer, the tobacco has been habitually retained in contact with that part." And in the same year, Dr. John Shew published a book entitled *Tobacco: Its History, Nature, and Effects on the Body and Mind* and asked a prophetic question: "I believe cancers . . . and tumors in and about the mouth will be found much more common among men than women. Since the former use tobacco much more generally than the latter, may not this be the cause?"

In 1859, a French physician named Bouisson presented his case study of sixty-eight patients with cancer of the oral cavity. Two-thirds of the cases were cancer of the lip, the others were cancer of the mouth, tongue, internal surface of the cheek, tonsil, and gum. The doctor reported that sixty-six of these patients smoked tobacco and one chewed tobacco. He also noted that cancer of the lip ordinarily occurred at the spot where the pipe or cigar was held.

Enter, Cigarettes

Again, the Bouisson and earlier reports were limited to cigar and pipe smokers, sniffers, and chewers. And the evidence was building that these particular forms of tobacco use were related to cancer. Ironically, just as Bouisson was indicting pipes, cigars, and chewing tobacco, cigarettes—"paper wrapped" tobacco, invented in the 18th century in Brazil—were first introduced into Britain by the troops from the Crimean campaign.

The early cigarettes were all rolled by hand and were not very popular items. First, due to the effort involved in producing them, they were available in limited quantities. Second, compared to pipes and cigars, cigarettes were considered "unmasculine." "Tell me what you smoke and I will tell you who you are," was the slogan of the day. A real man didn't smoke dainty hand-rolled weeds.

The invention of the cigarette-making machine in the 1870s changed all of that. And by 1885, because they were available and cheap, cigarettes were slowly being accepted in European and American society, and the prejudice against "tobacco rolled in paper" diminished.

The year 1885 also marked the death of General Ulysses S. Grant, an inveterate cigar smoker, from throat cancer. In the public mind, his cigar-smoking habit was associated with his military prowess. One of his greatest gifts from his admirers after his military victory over the South was a collection of eleven thousand cigars. Historical medical reports indicate that in his last months General Grant's deterioration and agony were such that he had to sleep sitting up to relieve the pressure and pain of his spreading malignancy.

By 1900, cigarettes had a firm grip on a small but growing proportion of American men. Not only were these "smokes" now readily available, but they offered the "advantage" of being mild enough to be inhaled. Furthermore, they fit in well with the fast pace of the new industrialism which characterized the first decade of this century. Pipes and cigars were for men of leisure, who had time to sip brandy and chat with each other about literature and world events. Cigarettes were for the busy man on the move, for men on the way up.

As cigarette smoking became more prevalent during the pre–World War I years, so did the indignant charges made by members of antitobacco league members. Cigarettes were again called "inventions of the devil" and, bound to ruin one's morals and at the same time indicted as "coffin nails," threats to health and well-being. The charges made against smoking were carried in books with titles like *The Use of Tobacco vs. Purity, Chastity and Good Health.* And the claims of the antitobacconists were so wrapped up in moral and ethical aspects of questions that the potential health problems were obscured.

Every time someone suggested prohibiting smoking, someone else sang its praises. In 1906, a doctor opined that modern women were drinking too much tea and he advised that they take up smoking as nicotine would counteract the stimulant in tea and prevent heart attacks. In 1911, when a French physician was asked about some documented cases of cancer among smokers, he responded that the cancer would have occurred anyway, the tobacco may have just determined the location. In 1918, *The New York Times* carried headlines which read "surgeons laud cigarettes" and a text which advised that servicemen be given a full supply as "the effect of the cigarette is wonderful."

In 1911 a new job was established, that of the "cigarette sampler." As the job description read, "All he has to do is give away an occasional pack with tact and discretion." The industry was on the move. It had a popular and potentially very lucrative product to sell, so why not solicit new customers, men who once they tried your product might well be with you for life?

There was certainly no reason to be concerned—even though, for the first time in American history, a significant portion of men (and a few, sly women) were regularly taking hot tobacco smoke into their lungs. Did anyone think of lung cancer then? No.

In 1912, Dr. I. Adler, commenting on U.S. disease patterns, wrote, "One point, however, *there is nearly complete consensus of opinion that primary malignant neoplasms of the lung are among the rarest forms of disease."* An average medical student being trained in this year never saw one case of lung cancer.

Cigarette sales were mounting steadily from the early 1900s until 1918, but World War I gave them a further boost. Basically, tobacco was used as a means of offering tranquility to the soldiers. General Pershing, Commander in Chief of the American troops in France, once cabled Washington saying, "Tobacco is as indispensible as the daily ration; we must have thousands of tons of it without delay." After the war, then, the praises of cigarettes were sung even louder. Said an article in the postwar *New York Times*, "To-bacco affords true enjoyment; it helps our organism over many dif-ficulties and over many cares and hardships leading to a depressed state. It satisfies thirst and hunger, as we learned during the war."

The years between 1920 and 1940 were those of the smoking heyday. Dr. John Harvey Kellogg's book, *Tobaccoism: How To-bacco Kills* (1922), which pointed to smoking as a cause of lip, throat, and mouth cancer, was not taken seriously. Even Miss Lucy Page Gaston and her associates, the outspoken represen-tatives of the Anti-Tobacco League which had all the vim and vigor of the Prohibition forces which succeeded in 1920 in passing the Twenty-third Amendment to prohibit the sale of alcoholic bever-ages, were having little effect. Miss Gaston wrote to President Harding, begging him not to smoke. Jovial cigarette lovers re-sponded by organizing a "cigarettes for Harding" campaign. Five years later, President Coolidge and Vice President Charles Dawes received similar requests. And of course they went on puffing.

In a land made dry by an Act of Congress, cigarettes offered a form of personal comfort which, for many, may have lessened the need to take advantage of the services of the local bootlegger.

Testimonials appeared frequently in the *Times*. "Smoked Sev-enty Years, Now Celebrating his Hundredth Birthday." "Doctor scoffs at charges that cigarettes interfere with health." "Smoking promotes health, MDs say. It increases the flow of gastric juices and contributes to evenness of temper." In October 1926, a front page *Times* story reported the findings of a Johns Hopkins profes-sor who had concluded that "smoking makes men more depen-dable," because it acts as a sedative. True, this expert conceded, "smoking does increase blood pressure slightly but so does telling a good joke." His conclusion? Smoking was good for you. People believed him.

Smoking readers probably found a 1929 *Times* story entitled, "Three Year Old Boy Is Regular Smoker" somewhat amusing. This particular child, one Maurice St. Pierre from Waterbury, Con-necticut, was said to have smoked two cigars, ten pipefuls, and a

pack of cigarettes each day. The story noted that he lit his own—
and that he had first taken up the habit when he was one-and-a-
half years old.

If you were not a cigarette smoker by 1935, you had a great deal
of resistance. The radio constantly sang the glories of cigarettes
and they came in all shapes, sizes, brands. The Prince of Wales
even came up with a half-sized cigarette which he recommended
as being ideal for puffing between dances.

Influential physicians testified in advertisements that "cigarettes
are kind to your throat" and opera singers claimed "we protect our
voices with Lucky Strikes." Models in costumes of Lucky Strike
green paraded up and down New York's Fifth Avenue smoking
cigarettes. And then came what may well be one of the most successful advertising campaigns in history, the slogan "Reach for a
Lucky Instead of a Sweet." Swiss chocolate sales plummeted and
the industry declared "the cigarette is a deadly enemy of chocolate." Weight-watching women looked with new interest to cigarettes. *Good Housekeeping* protested, "We're just old fashioned
enough to wish that women would not smoke." But the taboo on
female smoking began to lift. In 1934, Mrs. Franklin D. Roosevelt
was called "the first lady to smoke in public" and although by 1935
the habit was still much more popular with men, women were
gaining on them.

In 1935, 66 percent of men and 26 percent of women under
forty were cigarette smokers. The habit was almost unheard of at
the beginning of this same century.

The Evidence Mounts

Rumblings about serious health problems began to be heard
about 1930. But they were relatively innocuous ones. A German
researcher named Dr. Lickint reported that of some 4,000 patients
with bronchial cancer, 3,400 were men. He felt that sex difference
could be explained by smoking habits. Lickint went further: not
only did he think cigarette smoking increased the odds on developing lung cancer, but he thought that the products of burned tobacco might remain in the bladder and cause cancer there. (His

thoughts on this were confirmed some thirty-five years later.) A March, 1930, issue of the *Journal of the American Medical Association* (JAMA) carried a translated summary of his findings on the back page. But no one paid much attention to the Lickint hypothesis. Indeed on November 25, 1933, *JAMA* "after careful consideration of the extent to which cigarettes were used by physicians in practice," published its first advertisement for cigarettes (Chesterfield), a practice which was to continue for twenty years.

In 1931, commenting on his own clinical experience, Dr. Frederick Hoffman reported in the *Annals of Surgery* that "smoking habits unquestionably increase the liability to cancer of the mouth, the throat, the esophagus, the larynx, and the lungs." He was either ignored or contradicted.

In 1939, Dr. Phillip Matz, recalling that lung cancer was practically unheard of in 1912, wondered about why his autopsy records at the Veterans Hospital in Washington showed that deaths from lung cancer had increased 121 percent from 1931–37, while other cancers were up by 28 percent.

In 1939, Dr. F. Mueller, alarmed by the unprecedented increase in lung cancer in Germany reported in the chief cancer journal of his country (*Zeits fur Krebsforschung*) that of eighty-six patients with lung cancer, eighty-three smoked. Physicians and laymen scoffed at the reports. Maybe there was an increase in lung cancer, but maybe there wasn't. Maybe clinical techniques had improved so drastically since 1900 that doctors now were better able to diagnose this disease. Or if there indeed was more lung cancer, it was probably due to industrialization, tarred roads, or maybe even the apparent increase was a backlash from the serious epidemic of influenza that gripped this country in 1918. Certainly cigarettes, which offered so much pleasure to so many Americans, were not involved. Preposterous!

In February, 1936, Dr. Aaron Arkin and Dr. David Wagner of the University of Chicago made public their concern about the increase in lung cancer patients. "Ninety percent of all our patients were chronic smokers, and we believe that the inhalation of tobacco smoke may be an important factor in producing chronic irritation." At the International Cancer Congress in 1939, Dr. Alton Ochsner, a distinguished New Orleans surgeon, in conjunction with Dr. Michael DeBakey (who later was to gain fame in the field of heart surgery), declared, "It's our conviction that the increase in pulmonary carcinoma is due largely to the increase in smoking, particularly cigarette smoking which is universally associated with inhalation."

The advertisements in *JAMA* continued: "More Doctors Smoke Camels," "The Thoughtful Physician Sends Cigarettes to His Friends and Patients Over Seas." By the eve of World War II, the overwhelming percentage of American physicians (roughly 80 percent) like all other American males, were confirmed cigarette smokers. Certainly none of them were going to accept the idea that cigarettes were harmful on the basis of isolated reports. Nor were any of the smoking doctors going to foment concern in the public press. Indeed, very little was reported to American smokers in the late 1930s and mid-1940s about the possible relationship of cigarettes, cancer, and other diseases.

One exception is that of a report made by Dr. Raymond Pearl at Johns Hopkins. Studying the records of one hundred thousand heavy smokers (defined as over ten cigarettes a day) with those of one hundred thousand nonsmokers, he noted that 54 percent of the smokers died before sixty, while only 43 percent of nonsmokers did. His conclusions, which did make headlines, were that "smoking is associated with a definite impairment of longevity."

Pearl, a biostatistician, was strongly criticized by the medical press which retorted that "extensive scientific studies have proved that smoking in moderation by those for whom tobacco is not especially contraindicated does not appreciably shorten life."

In a 1948 editorial, *JAMA* went even further than that, stating that *"in all probability, more can be said in behalf of smoking as a form of escape from tension than against it."*

THE INDICTMENT

During that same year, Dr. Evarts Graham and Ernst Wynder, a student at the Washington University School of Medicine, were puzzling over the extraordinary rise in deaths from lung cancer.

Wynder thought that there was an important correlation between the growing popularity of cigarette smoking and lung cancer. Dr. Graham was unconvinced. He pointed out that there was also a correlation between rising lung cancer rates and the sale of nylon stockings.

But Graham did feel the subject was worth looking into. Besides, he had a personal interest in the subject: in 1933, he had become the first physician to successfully remove a human lung from a cancer victim (his patient was an obstetrician from Pittsburgh); he had seen firsthand clinical evidence of what some people were saying was the result of cigarette smoking.

Was it true what they said? He wanted to know. Dr. Graham himself was a smoker.

In 1949, Graham and Wynder accepted a grant from the American Cancer Society and began a study of 684 patients, almost all male, at the Washington University School of Medicine in St. Louis. What they found probably did not please Dr. Graham: 94 percent of these patients smoked cigarettes, some 3 percent pipes, and 3 percent cigars. Less than 2 percent of lung-cancer patients were nonsmokers or very light smokers.

But maybe that was because almost everyone these days was smoking. Maybe the findings didn't mean anything at all. The researchers took a look at a "control" group of hospital patients, that is, those *without* lung cancer: almost 15 percent of these men were nonsmokers. Furthermore, the number of heavy and chain smokers was twice as great among the lung-cancer patients as in the control group.

Dr. Graham and soon-to-be-Dr. Wynder reported their conclusions in a May, 1950 issue of the *Journal of the American Medical Association:* "Extensive and prolonged use of tobacco, especially cigarettes, seems to be an important factor in the inducement of bronchogenic carcinoma."

Dr. Graham made a concerted effort to stop smoking.

In September of 1950, the *British Medical Journal* carried an article entitled "Smoking and Carcinoma of the Lung," by Richard Doll, M.D., and A. Bradford Hill, Ph.D. These researchers began by explaining that they were puzzled by the "phenomenal" increase in deaths attributed to cancer of the lung. They noted that the pattern change in this form of death was the most striking one ever recorded by the Register General in England: in the quarter of a century between 1922 and 1947, the annual number of deaths from lung cancer increased roughly fifteenfold.

Their question was "why?" Doll and Hill considered two possible answers: (*a*) the effects of general atmospheric pollution from exhaust fumes of cars and the surface dust of tarred roads, coal fires and other industrial wastes; and (*b*) tobacco smoking.

They asked twenty hospitals in London to cooperate by notifying them of all patients admitted with carcinoma of the lung. These patients and a corresponding series of patients without lung cancer were interviewed. The results were startlingly similar to those announced just months before in the United States: of the men, less than 0.3 percent of lung cancer victims did not smoke; over 4 percent of those without lung cancer did not smoke.

(The fact that the overwhelming majority of men at the time were cigarette smokers accounts for the low percentage of nonsmokers in the non-lung-cancer group. From a statistical point of view, however, the results were and are highly significant.)

Medical scientists were beginning to take the subject of the cancer-producing potential of cigarettes more seriously. And the public press got interested. In 1950 *Reader's Digest* ran an article entitled "How Harmful Are Cigarettes?" pointing out the preliminary results of studies in progress, and raising some questions about the advisability of cigarette smoking. This article proved to be the first in an ongoing *Digest* attempt to bring the facts about the dangers of smoking to the attention of the public.[1] In contrast, also in 1950, *Coronet* featured an article. "The Facts About Cigarettes and Your Health," by authors who had "examined some fifty

1. It should be noted here that the *Reader's Digest* and *The New Yorker* are among the very few popular publications in the United States which now do not accept cigarette advertisements. The author has been severely limited in what she has been permitted to say about the health effects of cigarettes in many major magazines over the past few years, editors informing her that cigarette manufacturers would withdraw their much-needed accounts if critical comments were made about their products. It is thus no surprise that, although cigarette smoking is a major cause of death in this country, the majority of popularly-oriented publications ignore the subject.

pounds of medical books and journals" and concluded that the whole relationship between lung cancer and smoking was a hoax, specifically comparing it to the Orson Welles broadcast of an invasion from Mars.

Doll and Hill continued their studies in England. They gathered more information on lung-cancer victims. In 1952, they told the *British Medical Journal* that there was a definite association between lung cancer and smoking, especially cigarette smoking.

In 1952, the *Reader's Digest* carried an article entitled "Cancer by the Carton." The author informed his readers that as he started research on the piece, he was a two-pack-a-day smoker. He was now worried, enough so to limit himself to ten cigarettes a day.

"But we need proof," critics began to say. "We are not convinced by the mere statistical observation that lung cancer victims are more likely to be smokers than are people who don't have lung cancer. Instead of looking at people who already have the disease, why not follow a group of healthy smokers and see how many of them develop lung cancer?"

THE CONVICTION

And this indeed was going to be the next step. Researchers Doll and Hill in England gathered information from forty thousand physicians, thirty-five and over. They asked them, among other things, if they smoked. After the questionnaires were in, they kept track of the doctors for four-and-a-half years and when deaths occurred, the researchers obtained the death certificate. An analysis of this report showed that "mild smokers are seven times as likely to die of lung cancer as nonsmokers; moderate smokers are twelve times as likely to die of lung cancer as nonsmokers, immoderate smokers are twenty-four times as likely to die of lung cancer than nonsmokers."

The first "real proof" was in, and more was to follow. At the same time Doll and Hill were studying the English doctors, Drs. E. Cuyler Hammond and Daniel Horn were conducting a much more extensive study for the American Cancer Society. In their study, 22,000 volunteers conducted interviews in nine states. A total of more than 187,000 men were questioned about their smoking habits, and followed for forty-four months.

Dr. Hammond was a four-pack-a-day man. Dr. Horn smoked one pack a day. As the last IBM card snapped out of the computer, both of them switched to pipes.

What they found was enough to convince them: the total death rate, from all causes combined, was far higher among cigarette smokers than among nonsmokers or pipe and cigar smokers, and the death rate increased in direct relation to the number of cigarettes smoked.

The studies went on through the 1950s and early 1960s. The results were the same: cigarette smoking was a serious threat to health. "Well, maybe it's not the smoking, but something that cigarette users have in common," desperate smokers asked. A computer analysis by race, height, nativity, residence, occupation, education, alcohol consumption, and other criteria confirmed that the only significant difference between lung-cancer victims and those with higher than expected rates of heart disease, emphysema, bladder cancer, and other diseases, was cigarette smoking.

In 1957, the tide turned. The evidence could no longer be denied. The *New York Times* carried a front-page story on June 5, 1957 announcing, "Cigarette Smoking Linked to Cancer in High Degree."

One of the early researchers on the subject of cancer and lung cancer never read that story. Dr. Evarts Graham, finally personally convinced that cigarettes posed a serious health threat, gave them up completely in 1953. But for him it was too late. His colleague, Dr. Alton Ochsner, describes as "the saddest letter I ever got from anyone" the one he received from Graham two weeks before he died. In it he stated, "Because of our long friendship, you will be interested in knowing that they found that I have cancer in both my lungs. As you know, I stopped smoking several years ago but after having smoked as much as I did for so many years, too much damage had been done."

On June 1, 1961, the presidents of the American Cancer Society, American Heart Association, American Public Health Association, and National Tuberculosis Association wrote a letter to President John F. Kennedy, outlining some of the health dangers of cigarette smoking and pointing out that the resulting damage would be huge in terms of loss in life and economic productivity "unless appropriate health measures are taken." They requested a commission be established to look into the subject. On June 7, Surgeon General Luther K. Terry announced the formation of such a committee. And on January 11, 1964, the panel of ten physicians and scientists made their final report that "cigarette smoking is a health hazard of sufficient importance in the United States to warrant remedial action. . . . Cigarette smoking is causally related to lung cancer in men; the magnitude of the effect of cigarette smoking far outweighs other factors. The data for women, although less extensive, point in the same direction."[2]

HOW DO WE KNOW THAT CIGARETTES CAUSE CANCER?

A great many things about cancer are debatable because of lack of solid evidence, and differing interpretations. This is not so with regard to the impact of tobacco on risk of cancer of several sites. "It would be hard to find another subject so thoroughly and extensively investigated during the last 25 years," Dr. E. Cuyler Hammond, vice president of the American Cancer Society, has pointed out. Indeed it is remarkable how consistent all the evidence indicting cigarette smoking as a high-risk cancer factor has been.

It's worth emphasizing here that if just a *fraction* of the evidence implicating cigarettes in cancer were submitted in charges against just about any other substance, with the possible exception of

2. One member of the President's Committee was Dr. Louis Feiser, a cigarette smoker who even after he signed and submitted the report, told the press he "couldn't quit." One year after issuing the report, Dr. Feiser, aged sixty-six, was informed that he had a small tumor on his lung. He underwent surgery in September of 1965—and, as a result took the advice of his own Committee more seriously. He gave up cigarettes, telling the press, "While we were working on the report, I was convinced about the findings, but I thought I was healthier than the people involved in the report . . . after all, statistics are cold things. It's quite a different thing when it becomes a personal matter."

alcohol, there would have been no controversy at all. *If, for instance, the leaf in question were spinach, there would be one less vegetable in our garden.* But the subject was not spinach. The subject was a source of great emotional and physical dependency for a significant part of the world's population, one which had as much a grip on medical scientists as it did on the rest of the population. It was also a subject which had intense monetary implications, tobacco being a cash crop in sixteen states.

Cigarette smoking has been convicted on at least six counts as a cause of cancer.

1. *Cancer trends:* While lung cancer was an extremely rare disease at the beginning of this century, it is now the number one form of cancer death in American men.

   The twenty-five-year lag between the growth of cigarette popularity, and the upswing in lung cancer is consistent with our understanding of the cancer latency period. Similarly, the fact that there was a delay in the upswing of lung cancer in women is consistent with the fact that they began smoking later than did men.

2. *Human studies:* Not one statistical study has been reported that has not shown that patients with lung cancer smoke considerably more than patients who do not have lung cancer.

3. *Animal studies:* Cigarette smoke condensate has been shown to cause skin cancer in the rabbit, mouse, and rat.

   This is not surprising given that a series of carcinogens (see attached incomplete list) have been identified in tobacco smoke.

   Perhaps as a result of some innate wisdom, animals do not independently smoke. But experiments that have forced beagles to smoke have shown lung changes remarkably similar to those which are found in the lungs of smokers. In 1970, researchers who pumped cigarette smoke into the lungs of dogs demonstrated the development of a significant number of lung malignancies.

4. *Nonsmokers:* Lung cancer is a rare disease among nonsmokers. Religious groups, such as Seventh Day Adventists have very-low rates of lung cancer mortality or incidence.

5. *Ex-smokers:* Smokers who give up the habit reduce their odds of developing lung cancer. British physicians during the 1960s gave

up smoking to a greater extent than did the rest of the country's population. Over a period of the next ten years, the lung cancer rate for physicians declined 38 percent, while the rate went up 7 percent for the rest of the male population.

6. *Dose-response relationship:* Studies have been consistent in reporting that the more cigarettes an individual smokes, the more likely he or she is to develop lung cancer.

The question of *how* tobacco increases cancer risk is not yet answered. Perhaps the carcinogens in tobacco act directly on the target organs causing changes in the cell and the cell growth patterns. But the important point here is that we do not need a complete understanding of the mechanism of causation to reach a conclusion with regard to the dangers of tobacco. When John Snow implicated the Broad Street Pump, he was unfamiliar with the biological aspects of the cholera agent. But he did know the water from the pump was contaminated and should not be drunk. For the purposes of improving health, that was all that was necessary.

Just a Few of the Carcinogens
Identified in Tobacco Smoke

methylfluoranthenes
benz (a) anthracene
B-naphthylamine
dibenzo (c) carbazole
benzo (a) pyrene and
methylbenzo (a) pyrene
dimethylnitrosamine

WHAT ARE THE RISKS OF SMOKING?

Imagine that you have a severe weight problem, being fifty or sixty pounds heavier than you should be in terms of physical fitness. You've tried everything you can to lose the extra pounds but have had bad luck. What you need is some type of "miracle diet pill" which will make the fat just roll off. Then someone develops such a pill. It is inexpensive, acts quickly, is pleasant to use and has only one side effect: it *doubles* your risk of developing stomach cancer during your lifetime. In other words, it increases your risk of this type of cancer by 100 percent. Would you be interested? Presumably not.

The concept of "risk" is a difficult one to deal with. But when you look at the table below, try to keep in mind that hypothetical and undesirable "diet pill" which carries with it a frightening 100 percent increased risk of cancer. That risk pales compared to the risks that go with cigarette smoking.

We must emphasize here that by smoking a pack of cigarettes a day you would be assuming *all* of these risks at once. They are by no means mutually exclusive. Lung cancer, although it is the most talked-about risk associated with cigarettes, is not the only one. Indeed, although the emphasis in this book is on cancer, it is important to note that the most significant mortality risk of a smoker is *heart disease,* not any form of cancer. Thus, an enormously increased risk of heart disease, perhaps as much as 1,000 percent, must be added to the already grim tally.

As you can see, while some cancer risks are elevated by smoking pipes and cigars, these forms of smoking materials are considerably less hazardous than cigarettes.

TABLE 1

Percentage Increased Risk from Selected Causes of
Cancer among "Regular" Smokers[a]

	CIGARETTES	PIPE	CIGARS
Lung	684%	123%	115%
Mouth	890	200	300
Larynx	709	200	200
Esophagus	317	100	400
Bladder	100	0	0
Pancreas	169	0	0

[a] The figures on cigarettes, derived from an American Cancer Society survey, are based on the cancer mortality ratios among men with a history of smoking approximately a pack of cigarettes daily compared with men ages 45–64 who never smoked regularly. The figures on pipe and cigar smoking are averages derived from a number of studies.

TABLE 2

Percentage Increased Risk of Lung Cancer

CURRENT NUMBER OF CIGARETTES A DAY	PERCENTAGE OF INCREASED RISK
1–9	362%
10–19	762
20–39	1,369
40 or more	1,777
AGE BEGAN SMOKING	
25+	308
20–24	908
15–19	1,369
under 15	1,577

SOURCE: American Cancer Society survey of men aged 35–48 according to current number of cigarettes smoked per day.

Obviously, the more cigarettes you smoke and the earlier you started, the more at risk you are.

"Filters" and "Low Tar" Cigarettes

These risk factors are based on a combined group of filter and nonfilter tip, low, medium and high tar/nicotine smokers. It could be argued that they overstate the current problem because the majority of American smokers today use filter "low tar" cigarettes.

There is some validity to this argument. Recent analyses by Dr. E. Cuyler Hammond of the American Cancer Society indicate that lung cancer risks associated with low tar/nicotine cigarettes are some 10 to 30 percent lower; that at least some of the cancer-causing agents are either removed or prevented from entering the body. But the fact remains that nonsmokers have only 15 percent as many deaths from lung cancer as do those who smoke low tar–low nicotine cigarettes. Furthermore, it is now evident that those smoking between one and two packs of the low-tar/nicotine versions have a *higher* lung cancer death rate than those limiting themselves to one pack of high tar/nicotine cigarettes.

HOW TO PREVENT CANCER[3]

1. Cigarettes represent one of the two most serious cancer threats in the United States today (the other, diet, will be discussed in the next chapter). If you are sincere in your desire to avoid cancer, *you must give up cigarettes,* and preferably all forms of tobacco.

2. Do not fall into the delusion that goes, "Well, I don't have any other bad habits, so this one is OK." Cigarette smoking is one bad habit that can kill you, quickly and efficiently.

3. IF YOU MUST SMOKE,
—Use only "low tar" filter cigarettes.
—Limit yourself to not more than 8 cigarettes a day.
—Do not inhale deeply.
—Do not smoke the cigarette down to the filter line; put it out when you are halfway through.
—Do not drink alcoholic beverages, even at times when you are not smoking. As you will read in Chapter 5, alcohol enormously enhances the carcinogenic effect of tobacco.

3. You will find a full appendix in the back of this book which discusses techniques for kicking the habit.

4

DIET

"Whatsoever was the father of disease, an ill
diet was the mother."

George Herbert

CANCER AND DIET: MAKING THE LINK

Your eating patterns may play a major role in determining your
risks of developing certain types of cancer.

The bad news is that many epidemiologists now feel that in the
United States as much as 50 percent of cancers in women and 30
percent of all cancers in men are the result of an imprudent diet.
The good news is that, as a result, each of us has within our power
the capability of modifying our diet in a way which may reduce our
cancer risk by at least 30 percent.

International Variation

It is the fact that there are startling differences in the frequency
of various types of cancer around the world which lead us to believe that some environmental factor, most likely diet, is responsible.

As you can see from the table on page 75, countries like the
United States, Australia, Canada, and Denmark have relatively

high rates of cancer of the breast, prostate, colon[1] (and although not shown here, cancer of the uterine body and ovary)—and relatively low rates of stomach cancer. Countries like Costa Rica, Bulgaria, and Japan demonstrate the opposite pattern: high rates of stomach cancer, low rates of breast, prostate, colon cancer.

Two things are of interest here: First, the high rates for the breast, prostate, and colon generally go together. This at least suggests that they might have some common cause or causes. Second, countries with high rates of breast, prostate, and colon cancers generally have low rates of stomach cancer and vice versa.

This latter observation might mean either that the factor which causes the first group of cancer offers protection from stomach cancer or, more likely, that the causes are separate, and that, for instance, the United States is doing something "right" with regard to preventing stomach cancer and something "wrong" in relation to putting ourselves at high risk of breast, prostate, and colon cancer. On the other hand, the Japanese must be doing something "right" to explain their low risks of cancer of the colon, breast, and prostate and another something "wrong" in the stomach cancer area.

There are three ways that our diet could affect our cancer risk. First, we could have a dietary deficiency that either promotes cancer, or fails to offer some naturally occurring form of dietary cancer protection.

While it is true that certain gross deficiencies related to alcoholism, lack of dietary iron (Plummer-Vinson syndrome) and a few other nutrients do promote specific forms of carcinogenesis, these conditions occur only in extreme circumstances. Nutrient deficiency does not appear to play an important role in American cancer-death patterns.

Along the lines of a possible link between dietary deficiencies and cancer is the current interest in vitamin A-like compounds as a possible form of dietary cancer protection. Recently the National Cancer Institute began a test of a new drug, a synthetic chemical related to vitamin A, to see if it would have any effect on reducing

1. It is cancer of the colon, more than the rectum, which is of particular interest here because it is the much more common of the two and apparently is more influenced by diet; but reporting systems often group them together.

cancer incidence in one hundred people facing a high probability of bladder cancer. (As of this writing the results are not yet in.) These synthetic substances, called retinoids, are essential to the normal development of cells that line major organs and in animals have been shown to prevent precancerous changes. It is important to emphasize here that it is *not* vitamin A per se which is being tested for a possible cancer inhibition property, but rather a chemical related to it. Increasing your intake of vitamin A will not protect you from disease, unless you have some unusual and severe vitamin A deficiency. Indeed in high doses vitamin A can be toxic and particularly damaging to your liver.

Also related to the idea that there are certain substances which might offer protection from cancer, is the recently intensified popular fascination with laetrile, scientifically known as amygdalin, a cyanogenic glycoside found in the seeds of apricots, peaches, and plums. Not only has laetrile been promoted as a cure for cancer, but there are those who feel that including this substance in the daily diet will offer protection from the various forms of this disease. (When used as a diet supplement, laetrile is usually marketed as "vitamin B_{17}" [or "aprikern"], even though there is no such vitamin.) But contrary to the enthusiastic testimonials of those attempting to legalize laetrile (these individuals have been experiencing considerable success in state legislatures around the country), repeated studies at the Sloan-Kettering Institute in New York and elsewhere confirm that laetrile in any form neither cures nor prevents cancer.

The laetrile saga only underscores the reality that mythology is often more persistent than veracity.

Second, we could be eating some direct cancer-causing agent—a food additive or some contaminant, artificial or natural. As we'll discuss here and in a later chapter, there is no reason to believe that, except in extremely rare cases (one of which will be mentioned a few pages from now), that this is a factor.

Third, diet and cancer could be linked on the basis of specific excesses. It is this third possibility which will be the focus of attention in this chapter.

COLON, BREAST, PROSTATE[2]

Cancer of the breast is the leading cancer killer of American women. Cancer of the colon is the second leading cause of cancer death for both males and females. Prostate cancer is the third most common form of cancer death in men and, if it were not for cigarette smoking, it would be vying with colon cancer for the number one position among men.

Something has got to explain these very large differences in our rates of these cancers and those of, for instance, Japan.

Genetic arguments, that is, that certain nationalities are biologically "prone" to certain cancers, are not very convincing because people who move from a low risk country to a high risk country do not retain low risks. As has been pointed out above, second generation Japanese women here have a breast cancer pattern much the same as the national average, even though in their native land, this disease is relatively uncommon.

It could be argued that some other lifestyle factor is responsible for these differences, perhaps differential use of food additives, childbearing styles, or occupation. But there has never been any evidence to suggest that the minute amount of additives in our food could affect three such diverse sites. In the testing of additives in animal experiments, when problems are found they are concentrated on the liver or bladder, not the reproductive organs or colon. Additionally, the differences between countries have apparently existed for decades, and have not widened in the past fifty years when additive use has increased.

The differences in reproductive habits from country to country hardly seem enough to explain such great international variation. Furthermore, it is difficult to explain how childbearing could increase the incidence of cancer of the colon. Occupational differences are ruled out because the countries with the high rates manifest them for both males and females although, in the case of colon cancer, the mortality rates are consistently higher for men.

2. In general, the statements made about these three cancers also apply to cancer of the ovary and uterus. The discussion is limited to these three because they are among the most frequent causes of American cancer deaths.

There is one factor, however, which is the likely explanation for differences in the rate at which these diseases occur: while Japanese build their diets around fish, rice, and vegetables, limit their intake of fat to about 12 percent of total calories and cholesterol to 300 mg. a day or less, Americans eat rich red meats, eggs and dairy products with some 40 percent of dietary calories accounted for by fat, taking in on the average 600 mg, or more of cholesterol.

As shown in the chart below, other less affluent countries, and those following "non-Western diets" also have low rates of colon, breast, and prostate cancer. Countries with an eating pattern similar to ours have high rates of these diseases. For instance, Australia, Canada, and Denmark have similar disease statistics. Additionally, blacks who live in rural parts of the United States have a lower incidence of cancer of the colon than do blacks living in cities. Presumably rural dwellers are less affluent and eat less rich food.

It is this type of remarkably large difference in fat and cholesterol between dietary patterns A and B (see below) which may account for the vast differences in disease incidence between countries like Japan and the United States. As you'll see later in this chapter, the remedy in terms of dietary modification, is going to have to be rather great if it is going to have an effect.

Just to give you a specific example of variations in dietary fat and cholesterol, consider two extreme western-type menus, one rather spartan, one obviously too rich but in many respects an "all-American" diet.

The Evidence

The "proof" that an imprudent diet increases our odds on developing these three types of cancer (and probably other ones) is of a very different nature from the "proof" that linked cigarette smoking with lung cancer and other deadly diseases. The relationship between diet and cancer is almost exclusively based on international differences in the incidence of the disease and a worldwide correlation between intake of fat, particularly animal fat, and these three (and possibly other) carcinomas. In other words, the "causal

Selected Cancer Death Rates around the World 1970–71[a]

	Breast	Prostate Gland	Colon and Rectum		Stomach	
			MALE	FEMALE	MALE	FEMALE
Group #1						
United States	22	14	19	15	8	4
Australia	20	15	19	17	14	7
Canada	23	14	22	19	15	7
Denmark	25	13	18	13	17	9
Group #2						
Costa Rica	7	6	4	3	44	25
Bulgaria	10	6	8	7	32	19
Japan	4	2	9	6	62	33

[a] Annual age-adjusted death rate per 100,000 population.
SOURCE: World Health Statistics Annual 1970–71.

	A	B

Breakfast:	juice
	cereal (cornflakes)
	skim milk
	coffee, tea, with lemon
	  or non-dairy creamer
		2 eggs
		bacon
		toast (2 pieces) with
		  butter
		glass of whole milk

Lunch:	piece of baked chicken salad dressing iced tea	cheeseburger french fries milk shake cherry pie
Dinner:	fruit cup swordfish with lemon rice broccoli margarine bread angel food cake tea or coffee	sirloin steak mashed potatoes with butter bread and butter chocolate cake
Approximate total dietary fat:	35 gm.	178 gm.
Approximate total cholesterol:	165 mg.	900 mg.

link" between diet and cancer is not anywhere near as strong as are other links in the etiology of human malignancy.[3]

But if the relationship is a valid one, it should hold up under cross-examination. For instance, is it true that groups of individuals living in the United States but following a low fat dietary pattern have lower rates of these types of malignancy? Yes, it is. Mormons and Seventh Day Adventists who use fatty foods relatively infrequently, have lower than expected death rates from cancer of the breast, prostate, and colon.[4] Is there any correlation between other diseases which are linked with fat intake and these forms of cancer? Yes, there is. For instance, countries which have a high rate of heart disease, which we've known for years can be promoted by too much fat and cholesterol-rich foods, also have a high rate of colon cancer.

Is there other human evidence? Actually, there is a great deal of it. Breast cancer is unusually common among Jewish women in New York City, as compared with women of other ethnic backgrounds. In Israel, cancer of the breast is common among that portion of the Jewish population coming from Europe, and uncommon among Jews coming from Asia and Africa. A rich versus a moderate or low-fat diet may be a key factor.

And what about in the laboratory? Is there any evidence there? Yes, again. A high-fat diet enhances the development of both spontaneous and chemically induced breast tumors in experimental animals.

FATS, HORMONES AND CANCER

Breast and Prostate

How could an overly rich diet increase one's chances of cancer? All the answers are not in yet, but there are some very solid leads.

3. The preliminary nature of this diet-cancer link must be emphasized. Certainly the evidence on high fat diets favoring cancer development is not strong enough to warrant a government policy statement (as has been made with regard to tobacco). The epidemiological association between overnutrition and cancer is presented here with the hope that the reader will interpret it critically and consider making moderate—not drastic—modifications in his dietary patterns.

4. Mormons in Utah have only 60 percent to 75 percent of the national average rate of cancer. Seventh Day Adventists have slightly more than half of the national cancer death rate.

A high-fat, high-cholesterol diet from childhood on may over-stimulate our endocrine system, producing much the same effect that one would get running a Volkswagen on high-octane airplane fuel. (But exactly how hormones relate to breast and prostate cancer is difficult to demonstrate. For one thing, a hormone level at age 55 may not be relevant in explaining hormonal risk factors to which a person was exposed at age 25.) Possibly when we eat a great deal of cholesterol-rich or fatty foods, our bodies respond by releasing increased amounts of hormones, setting into action a chain of events which alter the biochemical balance, leaving the breasts and prostate, and possibly other organs, less immune to disease and favoring the growth of cancerous tumors. We may be biochemically unable to metabolize such dietary excesses.

Since almost all mammary tumors require hormones at some point in their development (particularly the hormones estrogen and prolactin), it seems most likely that dietary fat exerts its effect on the breast (and presumably other organs as well) via the endocrine system rather than by a direct effect on mammary tissue itself. Dr. Ernst Wynder and his associates at the American Health Foundation have proposed, as a working concept, that high levels of dietary fat induce increased levels of serum prolactin,[5] thereby stimulating the development of preexisting malignant breast lesions.

We do not know right now if the increased hormone production is the *cause* of these types of cancer. Perhaps the step-up in hormone production serves to initiate or promote another cancer-causing agent. But whatever the mechanism, the implications are clear.

Colon

Here again is a situation where an apparent cause-effect association of fat intake and disease, bringing together endocrinology and nutrition exists, but without a full biological explanation of the way it all happens.

It's been suggested that the fat intake of our diet, which nor-

5. A more detailed discussion of prolactin and its possible role in breast cancer can be found in the chapter dealing with sexual factors in cancer etiology.

mally parallels cholesterol consumption, increases bile production and flow. Preliminary studies have shown that the feces of individuals on high-fat diets contain more bile acids than do those on a low-fat diet. Colon cancer patients have a higher content of neutral steroids and bile acids—by-products of cholesterol—in their stools than do controls. One current working hypothesis is that cholesterol is a carcinogen and bile acids are tumor promoters. Again, we have a case of excessive dietary fat overstimulating the body. It is possible that some of the metabolites of this excessive bile acid are capable of causing cancer. Alternatively, the large amounts of fat we eat may act directly on the bacteria normally present in the colon, causing them to produce carcinogens, specifically the steroid hormones estradiol and estrone. Estradiol and estrone, which are fractions of the hormone estrogen, regularly produce tumors in animals and are suspected of playing a role in a number of forms of human cancers. Indeed, if the intestinal bacteria do produce estrogens in the presence of fat and cholesterol, it is possible that breast cancer and other diseases, as well as colon cancer, may be promoted in this manner.

Fiber

No discussion of the cause and prevention of colon cancer is complete without mentioning fiber (sometimes known as "roughage" or "bulk"), that modern-day fountain of youth.

Dr. Denis Burkitt, a surgeon who spent many of his years of medical practice in Africa, and after whom one rare form of malignancy (Burkitt's Tumor) is named, is convinced that the lack of dietary fiber is a major cause of five common diseases in developed countries, among them cancer of the colon. He and others have emphasized that a high fiber diet, as opposed to one which consists mainly of highly processed foods, offers protection from colon cancer by increasing stool volume and promoting a more rapid "transit time" for the feces. He suggests that when the bowel is exposed to stools for a longer period of time, the organ is irritated and possibly exposed to potentially cancer-causing agents for a prolonged period.

At this point, however, the "high-fiber diet" idea remains just one of many hypotheses. Americans often look for quick solutions and thus are now stuffing themselves with bran. But it is risky to attribute such a complex disease to one cause, given that there are some serious gaps in the "fiber-cancer" theory. For example, there is no increased risk of colon cancer in any individuals who chronically suffer from constipation, an observation which casts doubt on the "transit time" theory. Furthermore, experiments with diet modification in animals does not support the notion that high-fiber diets offer protection from cancer. Additionally, there is no correlation between fiber content of foods and the incidence of colon cancer in countries around the world. But there *is* such a correlation for fat ingestion. Perhaps people eating a great deal of bran, and high-in-fiber vegetables and fruit simply have little room for fatty foods. So the high-fiber recommendation might be right for the wrong reasons.

Whether or not it offers a direct protective effect for cancer of the colon and other diseases, bran and other crude cereals are an excellent—and delicious—contribution to a well-balanced diet.

Cancer and General Caloric Intake

Because such a large portion of our calories consists of fat, it is difficult to study the cancer-causing effects of overeating and obesity per se. Right now our emphasis is on fat intake, but it should be noted that obesity itself, as well as fat consumption, has been linked with an increased risk of cancer of the body of the uterus in women.

STOMACH

Having acknowledged that we are apparently doing something wrong in terms of diet and its effect on certain types of cancer, it's time to point out that we are doing something right in reducing stomach cancer odds. There has been a steady decrease in the incidence of this disease (by more than 50 percent in twenty-five years, for both men and women). Our death rate from stomach cancer is one-third of that thirty years ago.

Let's start by asking what is it about the Japanese culture that could explain that their male rate of stomach cancer is 62 while ours is 8? One obvious difference is the way they prepare and store their food.

Eating in Japan

Japanese love to use salt—lots of it. Salty foods, such as soybean paste (miso), soybean sauce (shoyu), salted pickles (shiozuke), and small fish, shellfish, or seaweed boiled with soybean sauce (tsuku-dani) are eaten as side dishes to complement boiled white rice. The salt content of these foods is about 10 percent for soybean paste, 18 percent for soybean sauce, 10 to 13 percent for salted pickles and about 3 to 20 percent (as a common preservative) for raw or dried salted fish. And that's a lot of salt.

Additionally, polycyclic aromatic hydrocarbons, standard animal carcinogens, and possible human carcinogens, may be finding their way into traditional Japanese meals. The strongest correlation between dietary polycyclics and human cancer is that all populations consuming a great deal of smoked fish seem to run a high risk of stomach cancer.

A favorite Japanese fish preparation technique (for instance, in preparing teriyaki) involves salting and drying it and then broiling it until it is burned black. Sometimes rice is prepared this way too. Cold rice can be formed into balls and baked. The surface of the rice ball is burned slightly black and it becomes as hard as glass. Apparently the Japanese enjoy the burned salty taste and appreciate the chewy sensation of the food.

Rice, the great staple of the Japanese diet, sometimes makes up as much as 50 to 60 percent of the food consumed. Some recent unsettling reports indicate that some Japanese rice is flavored with a talc substance very closely related to asbestos, a known human carcinogen.

In addition to their consumption of salt, "burned" substances, and possibly contaminated rice, it's been suggested that the high rate of stomach cancer in Japan can be explained by their frequent use of very hot dishes and beverages, factors that might enhance the effects of carcinogens in the food. For instance, in some districts of Japan where the stomach cancer rate is extraordinarily high, a very hot rice gruel (chagayu) is eaten every morning. Japanese sake, made from boiled white rice to which a fungus is added, is usually drunk warm—sometimes very hot. Hot sake causes a burning feeling in the esophagus and stomach.

Other possible leads which may help explain stomach cancer prevalence in Japan are that the known animal carcinogen, bracken fern, an asparaguslike vegetable, is frequently used in salads, and their fish may have naturally high levels of nitrate which may convert internally to nitrite, eventually forming substantial amounts of cancer-causing nitrosamines.

Other Countries with High Rates of Stomach Cancer

Obviously the dietary pattern for Japan cannot fully explain why other countries, for instance, Costa Rica and Bulgaria, have such elevated rates of this disease. So what are *they* doing wrong? Again, food preparation, particularly the use of smoking as a preservative and possibly primitive and health-threatening means of food storage which allow the food to become contaminated. It is also possible as is explained below that it is the *lack* of certain chemicals in the diet which may account for the high rate of stomach cancer in some countries.

Eating in the U.S.

For a number of reasons, our diet or food-processing procedures are apparently protecting us from stomach cancer. It would be useful to determine what we are doing right so that when we modify our diets to lessen our chance of cancer of the breast, colon, and prostate, we don't sacrifice what has been helpful to us or, worse, pick up some new bad habits.

Although at this point it remains unproven, there is reason to believe that the declining rate of stomach cancer in this country is, in part due to the use of antioxidants in our diet, specifically the food additives BHA and BHT (Butylated Hydroxyanisole and Butylated Hydroxytoluene) which are used widely in oil, margarine, bakery products and other substances. These, and other antioxidants have been shown to inhibit cancer in laboratory animals, and their use in this country parallels the decline in stomach cancer.

The interest in antioxidants and cancer prevention is being extended to include antioxidants other than BHA and BHT. It has recently been suggested that it's the relatively high intake of dietary selenium in Japan (Japanese eat two to four times as much of this trace element as we do, generally getting it in their grains, vegetables, and fish), which plays a protective role in breast cancer.

In addition to the use of antioxidants, we have a relatively effective food storage system in this country. Food has a minimal chance to become contaminated. Additionally, smoked, highly spiced, and salted foods are not a regular part of our diet. Neither are grilled foods. There is no reason to suspect that an occasional charcoal-broiled hamburger will introduce substantial amounts of carcinogens into our system. If you are concerned about a cancer threat at a barbecue, probably the beef (if it is a cut with a high-fat content) should concern you more than the grilling.

Interestingly enough, while our country as a whole has a very low rate of stomach cancer, there are certain "hot spots" with unusually high rates of this disease. There is an impressive cluster of stomach cancer in rural counties in the north-central region of the nation (Minnesota, Dakotas, Michigan and Wisconsin). Concentrated in these areas are people of Russian, Austrian, Scandinavian, and German descent. Susceptibility of these ethnic groups to stomach cancer would be compatible with the fact there is a high incidence of this type of tumor in their native lands.

This type of clustering provides another clue. The dietary patterns of these areas are now being intensively studied. Already, however, a common theme is emerging: highly spiced, smoked food.

Cancer-Causing Agents?

The emphasis here has been on overeating, particularly too much fat and cholesterol, as the cause of a number of different types of cancers. We've acknowledged that in some circumstances particular deficiencies may be involved. But interestingly, when most people think of diet being "linked with cancer" they think of the possibility that we are eating cancer-causing agents. The subject of food additives, pesticide residues, and their possible involvement in human cancer will be the subject of Chapter 11. But here it is important to acknowledge again that there are very, very few dietary chemicals which are known—or even suspected—to cause cancer in humans. One exception to that statement is the mold aflatoxin.

The Shangaans, a tribe in Swaziland, Africa, are fond of the groundnuts that proliferate in the lowlands of their region. They grind the shelled nuts in a wooden mortar and pestle and the resulting rather oily and sticky powder is sprinkled on food as a condiment, much in the same way we use salt and pepper. They also add it to the rich soups they consume regularly. Enough is prepared for about a week and the groundnut mash is stored for later use.

Among the Shangaan males, liver cancer is the most common form of cancer.

In the Netherlands, a group of workers whose task it was to extract oils from peanuts were found to have rates of cancer and liver disease at a rate of three times that of a matched control group.

In England in 1961, thousands of turkey poults, ducklings, and chicks died of acute liver disease. About the same time, in the Northwest United States, thousands of rainbow trout, the favorite game fish of the region, died as the result of liver tumors.

What the Shangaans, Dutch workers, turkey poults, ducklings, chicks, and rainbow trout had in common was exposure to nuts that were contaminated with the natural carcinogenic molds known as *aflatoxins* (*Aspergillus flavus*).

Aflatoxins are suspicious enough molds so that a concerted effort is made in this country to keep them out of our food. Peanut products are regularly inspected and, on occasion, batches from other countries are rejected.[6]

Aside from aflatoxins, only two other substances have ever been classified on the basis of human studies as "possible dietary human carcinogens": bracken fern, the asparaguslike vegetable which we mentioned is often part of the Japanese diet. Bracken has been shown to cause bone marrow damage and urinary tumors in cattle fed the whole plant or extracts. The fact that it is eaten in Japan where the stomach cancer death rate is so very high at least suggests it may play a possible role there.

Nitrosamines, which are naturally forming chemicals that can develop on vegetables such as maize or spinach (the conversion process is one from the chemical nitrate to nitrite to nitrosamines) has been suggested as a possible direct carcinogen to account for the high rate of cancer of the esophagus in parts of Africa. In these areas, a maize beer, which may be contaminated with natural nitrosamines, may be involved. Again, the link of nitrosamines with human cancer is now only speculative. The possible dangers of nitrites and nitrosamines will be discussed in a later chapter.

EATING FOR GOOD HEALTH

As Rene Dubos summarized it, we are suffering from a severe case of "malnutrition of the affluent."

What is the remedy for our overconsumption of cholesterol-rich fatty foods? On this public health and nutrition experts are in unanimous accord: switch to a more prudent diet.

The original Prudent Diet was first introduced in the late 1950s by Dr. Norman Jolliffe, who started the Diet and Coronary Disease Project (popularly known as the "anticoronary club") at the New York City Health Department's Bureau of Nutrition. The

6. Given the current popularity of the "zero tolerance" principle and food additive laws which prohibit the use of even trace amounts of an additive which has been shown to cause cancer in humans or animals, it is interesting to note that the FDA has now set tolerances for the presence of aflatoxins in foods. In other words, they apparently feel that small amounts of this natural carcinogen are either acceptable or unavoidable. Aflatoxins are not subject to the Delaney Clause because they are not food additives.

diet is aptly described as "a way of eating consistent with the American dietary pattern while avoiding an excess of empty calories, saturated fat, and food cholesterol."

The "prudent diet" we will discuss here as a means of reducing cancer risks is not exactly the same as the Jolliffe Prudent Diet. It does stress a favorable balance of nutrients, and meets the needs for protein, minerals, and vitamins, increasing the use of polyunsaturated fats as did the Jolliffe plan.

But eating prudently to avoid cancer goes further than this. It stresses the reduction of *all* fatty foods—of animal and vegetable origin.

It does not recommend that you become a vegetarian (if you choose to, and make sure your diet is well-balanced, that's fine), nor does it suggest you totally eliminate all fats, or give up beef. It is based on moderation, a varied diet, and a recognition that some foods have very high levels of polyunsaturated fats, saturated fats, cholesterol, or all of these. But, on the other hand, compared to what most Americans eat, it does represent a moderate change. Specifically it calls for *cutting in half* the amount of cholesterol and fat that most of us consume.

In recent years, epidemiologists have begun to detect some payoff in the area of heart disease. Premature deaths among men from heart attacks do appear to be declining, and at least part of that decline can probably be attributed to more prudent eating habits (although a significant portion of the decline is likely the result of a diminishing popularity of cigarette smoking). With some extra effort and a further cutback in fat and cholesterol intake, we might see the current breast cancer situation in this country improve. We should now be encouraging various segments of the food industry to help solve the problem at the site of origin: by devising a means of producing eggs which are naturally low in cholesterol, developing strains of animals that convert higher proportions of their feed to protein rather than fat, experimenting with new high-quality vegetable proteins, producing more foods with less fat and more water, and further encouraging manufacturers of baked goods to substitute polyunsaturated fats for the traditional saturated variety. But in the meantime there are some specific dietary guidelines we should consider.

HOW TO PREVENT CANCER[7]

Step Number 1: *Limit your use of egg yolks* and other cholesterol-rich foods. Scientists at the American Health Foundation recommend that you should consume *no more than 300 mg. of cholesterol each day,* preferably much less. The fact that one egg yolk alone has about 235 mg. of cholesterol gives you an idea about how easy it is to far exceed that limit with an egg and bacon breakfast, a cheeseburger for lunch, and a sizzling steak to top off the evening.

In terms of practical manu planning, consider limiting your consumption of "visible egg yolks" (that is, not counting eggs which are used in baked products and elsewhere where they are not immediately evident) to two to four per week. Continue to buy eggs, just throw out the yolks. The whites are full of nutrients and do not threaten your health.

Many recipes requiring eggs can be satisfactorily prepared using egg whites with added polyunsaturated vegetable oils. Additionally, a number of new "egg substitutes" (like "Second Nature" and "Egg Beaters") offer you an excellent breakfast alternative. "Second Nature" also offers the advantage of having half the calories of natural eggs.

In meal planning to keep your cholesterol below 300 mg. a day, note that while chicken, fish, and veal are lower in cholesterol than other sources of protein, they do have quite a bit themselves. On the other hand, products of plant origin, such as fruits, vegetables, cereals, grains, legumes, nuts, and oils have no cholesterol.

Step Number 2: *Cut back significantly on all high-fat foods. Keep your intake of fats below 80 grams a day. Specifically, limit fat consumption to thirty to thirty-five percent of your total daily calories. Each gram of fat contributes 9 calories. (see Appendix II for estimates of fat content of commonly eaten foods).*

Step Number 3: *Cut back significantly on your consumption of all fats,* particularly whole-milk dairy products, oils and fatty meats.

Use more veal, chicken, turkey, and fish, but don't feel you must eliminate or even cut back drastically on beef, pork, and

7. See Appendix II for some specific information on the cholesterol and fat levels of various foods, and for some tips on eating prudently.

lamb. Continue to use these meats but choose lean cuts only, *trim off all visible fat* and make sure the serving sizes are small. You need not go to extremes in avoiding fats and oils. But use some common sense. If you are making a meat sauce, pour off the fat once the meat is cooked and before you add other ingredients. Avoid using fatty meat drippings for gravies.[8] Use fried foods sparingly. Take advantage of the low-fat oleomargarines, cheeses, mayonnaises.

Include fish at least two or three times weekly.

Use skim milks and cheeses instead of whole-milk products.

Step Number 4: *Eat many more fruits and vegetables,* particularly green leafy vegetables. Plan at least one "no meat or fish" meal each week.

Step Number 5: *Include more cereals,* especially crude cereals and enriched rices, in your diet.

Step Number 6: *Limit your consumption of rich, creamy, or chocolate desserts.* For snacks, in addition to fruits and vegetables, try gelatin, water ices, sherbert, angel food cake, almond macaroons, sponge cake.

It has been said that in the end the patient, in this case, the human race, will die of civilization. Obviously, one aspect of spreading civilization has been a dangerously excessive diet. But the problem can be remedied, and the patient can be saved.

8. To cut back on fat ingestion here, pour all the drippings into a container, place in freezer for 15 minutes, then spoon off fat which has hardened on top.

5

ALCOHOL

"Drink not the third glass, which thou canst
not tame,
When once it is within thee."

George Herbert
The Temple, 1633

TO YOUR HEALTH!

There is no good evidence that alcohol alone causes cancers in either animals or humans. But there is reason to believe that excessive amounts of it do, perhaps in some indirect manner, increase the risk of a number of types of human cancers.

Ethyl alcohol has been part of the human diet for at least 1,000 years. But it was only after the association was made between tobacco and lung cancer that attention was given to other personal habits, like drinking patterns and the possible role they might have in carcinomas.

Right away, the association of spirit consumption and malignant disease was a difficult one to establish. Animal studies showed nothing. Even at very high dose-levels (20 percent alcohol in their drinking water for a prolonged time) alcohol does not cause an increase in tumors.

Studies of human drinking patterns to some degree have been thwarted by the fact that people do not tell the truth—or perhaps they just don't remember—how much they consume. Unless you carefully measure each drink, keep track of how many you have, and have about the same amount each time you drink, your response would be only an estimate. If you drink a lot, the estimate would likely be on the low side. Beyond that, the use of alcohol and tobacco are so intertwined (one study of alcoholics showed that over 90 percent smokes cigarettes) that it is usually difficult to distinguish which factor is responsible for the resulting damage.

And added to all this confusion are some very strong personal feelings about the subject. If you are a teetotaling researcher you may have different ideas than if you enjoy a couple of martinis before dinner each night. Much like the case of cigarettes, research on the topic of alcohol and cancer appears to have been inhibited by our society's great fondness for cocktails, highballs, wine, and beer. Perhaps it's simply human nature to resist information which suggests that something you like is harmful.

"TOO MUCH" AND CANCER

Definitions of "heavy drinking" vary but, on the average, most studies of alcohol and cancer draw the line at two or three ounces of absolute alcohol a day.

If each day you drink more than three ounces, the equivalent of three drinks each with about 2 ounces of 80 proof liquor, five 5-ounce glasses of table wine, or six 8-ounce glasses of beer, you would be considered to be a heavy drinker. If you do not drink every day but imbibe only on weekends or go on "binges" which average that on a daily basis, you would also be in this category.

Unfortunately, in our discussion of the possible role alcohol may have on increasing your risks of cancer, we are unable to indicate the exact risk factor by amount consumed. We cannot tell you that if you have four strong drinks each day you will increase your odds by x percent.

The reason that our information here is incomplete is that the whole subject is so new. For instance, the American Cancer Society's book, *Cancer: A Manual for Practitioners,* published in 1970, does not mention that alcohol may play a role in any form of this disease. Similarly, the first Public Health Service *Special Report to Congress on Alcohol and Health,* published in 1971, never mentioned cancer. (The Second Report, issued in 1974, did. Indeed, it dedicated a whole section to the topic.)

But although our knowledge about the role that alcoholic beverages alone play in cancer is still quite sketchy, right now there *is* evidence, based on human studies, that alcohol in some manner elevates cancer risk at several body sites. Thus alcohol cannot be passed off as a "hypothetical risk." The results of these limited studies deserve our attention.

The Esophagus

The esophagus is the first portion of the gastrointestinal tract to be exposed to ingested alcohol.

A number of studies indicate that the risk of esophageal cancer is some seventeen times greater among alcoholics and twice as high among bartenders. In both the United States and France, there seems to be a good correlation by geographic area, with a steep increase in esophageal cancer mortality rates with increasing amounts of distilled spirits sold per capita.

Cigarette smoking could play some role in these increased risks, but because the relationship between cancer of the esophagus and heavy drinking can be identified from records fifty or more years ago when cigarette smoking was not yet a widespread habit, and because the limited studies which have attempted to remove the effect of smoking have indicated a higher esophageal cancer incidence among drinkers, there is reason to believe that, through some yet to be established mechanism, ingestion of significant amounts of alcohol will increase your risk of this disease.

As we've already mentioned, the subject simply has not been studied as much as has cigarette smoking and relative risks have not been scientifically established. But, as a working figure, you might consider that by drinking more than five or six ounces, or just slightly more of 80 proof liquor each day, or the equivalent in wine and beer, you may increase your odds on developing cancer of the esophagus by two or three times, that is by 100 to 200 percent. If you drink considerably more than that, your risk would be at least proportionally greater. As we'll mention below, the extent of the risk may depend on the type of alcohol you use, and will definitely depend on whether or not you smoke cigarettes.

Alchohol probably plays a significant role in the etiology of cancer of the esophagus in this country. But unlike tobacco use, which can explain the distribution of lung cancer around the world, alcohol explains only a small amount of esophageal cancer. For instance, in parts of Iran where there is no large amount of alcohol consumed, the rates from this type of cancer are extraordinarily high.

Oral Cancer

Alcohol and tobacco are both well known risk factors for cancer of the mouth and pharynx, together considered responsible for approximately 75 percent of all cancers of the oral cavity in American men. Here, especially, we have the problem of separating out the two factors to see which is more important, what proportion of the risks are attributable to each.

The limited studies which have taken cigarette smoking into account suggest that heavy drinkers who do not smoke increase their risks of various forms of oral cancer by two to three times, that is by 100 to 200 percent; certainly the risk would be greater for very heavy drinkers.

Larynx

Laryngeal cancer occurs much more frequently in alcoholics than nonalcoholics. Although this increase may be partly due to heavy smoking, the rates of laryngeal and lung cancers in alcoholics differs dramatically from the proportions generally seen in nonalcoholic heavy smokers. This suggests that alcohol alone may play a role here. Again, a working "risk factor" of two to three times greater probability of developing larynx cancer seems appropriate here.

Liver

Alcoholics with cirrhosis of the liver have a much higher than expected rate of liver cancer. Whether or not this observation has any relevance in terms of liver cancer risk to the individual who has three or four cocktails a day is unknown. Because it is the liver which has the primary responsibility for detoxifying alcohol, it seems at least plausible that a constant massive bombardment of that organ with liquor might cause its tissues to change in a way which might favor carcinogenic growth. But the evidence which definitely links moderate, or even heavy but nonalcoholic, drinking patterns with increased incidence of liver cancer, has not been gathered yet, possibly because this form of malignancy is relatively rare in our country.

Other Cancers

There is no firm evidence which suggests that alcohol consumption will affect your chances of developing cancer of the rectum, stomach, pancreas, or prostate gland. Several investigators have postulated a relationship between cancer of the colon and heavy beer drinking, but the results here have been conflicting.

HOW ALCOHOL MAY INCREASE CANCER RISK

Nutritional Factors

If you regularly consume a great deal of alcohol, you may well have a very unbalanced diet, often because after a few drinks you have no appetite for food. A number of vitamin and mineral deficiencies have been found in alcoholics, particularly a lack of thiamine, folic acid, magnesium, iron, and zinc. A disease known as Plummer-Vinson syndrome, which often sets the stage for cancers of the mouth, pharynx, and esophagus, has been linked to deficiencies of Vitamin B complex and iron. It is possible then that it is a poor diet, as opposed to the alcohol itself, which may leave heavy drinkers susceptible to cancers of a number of sites.

Tissue Effect

Given that alcohol is a pharmacologically strong substance, it is possible that its prolonged contact with the tissues of the mouth, esophagus, and liver may irritate other areas, bringing about significant cellular changes which allow carcinogens to thrive. By decreasing saliva volume, alcoholic beverages may leave the tissues of the esophagus particularly exposed.

Immune System

One cancer theory states that we are constantly being exposed to thousands if not millions of potentially carcinogenic substances in our environment, but in 99 percent or more of the cases, our bodies reject them courtesy of an elaborate immunological system. Alcohol may affect one or more of the mechanisms of our host defense system, leaving us vulnerable to whatever cancer-causing agents we encounter.

A Contaminant?

Perhaps it is not the alcohol itself which increases cancer risk, but rather a contaminant of the drink. For instance, fusel oil, a by-product of distillation and a possible carcinogen, is found in varying quantities in different liquors. Fusel oil, and other congeners, that is those substances which give liquor their taste and color, are found in large amounts in bourbon and are nearly absent in vodka.

In Puerto Rico where there is a high rate of head and neck cancer, there is also a high consumption of "moonshine" rum which contains far more fusel oil than the commercial rum produced under government control. In parts of Africa where the esophageal cancer rate is very high, the locally brewed maize beer is thought to be contaminated with nitrosamines, natural substances which have been shown to be highly carcinogenic in animals. In France, which has an overall elevated risk of cancer of the esophagus, the rate fluctuates from area to area, being highest in the northwestern regions where the main alcoholic beverage produced is apple brandy rather than wine.

We do not know very much about the nonalcoholic substances in the whiskey, beer, and wine we drink in the United States, but if there is something to this theory, vodka on the rocks, perhaps with a twist of lemon, would seem about the safest alcoholic drink.

Cocarcinogen

There is good reason to believe that alcohol, rather than being a direct cancer-causing agent itself, acts as a cocarcinogen, that is it

Percentage Increased Risk for Oral Cancer According to Level of Exposure to Alcohol and Smoking

	Cigarettes per Day		
ALCOHOL[a]	LESS THAN 20	20–39	40 OR MORE
None	52%	43%	143%
Less than .4 ounces	67	218	225
.4–1.5 ounces	336	346	721
More than 1.5 ounces	313	859	1,450

[a] This is pure alcohol. 1.5 ounces would be the equivalent of 3.75 ounces of 80 proof liquor.

SOURCE: Adapted from Rothman, K. J. and Keller, A. Z. "The Effect of Joint Exposure to Alcohol and Tobacco on Risk of Cancer of the Mouth and Pharynx", *J. Chron. Dis.* 25:711, 1972.

promotes cancer in conjunction with another carcinogen. The most serious, indeed deadly, example we know where alcohol acts as a cancer promoter is when it teams up with cigarettes.

If you smoke two packs of cigarettes a day, you assume a 143 percent greater risk of developing cancer of the oral cavity than does a person who does not smoke cigarettes. If, however, in addition, you have just two alcoholic drinks a day, your risk skyrockets to almost 1,500 percent. Presumably alcohol enhances the effects of tobacco at other sites too, particularly the esophagus, and larynx, but not the lung simply because alcohol does not come in contact with that organ.

HOW IMPORTANT IS THE CANCER THREAT FROM ALCOHOL?

If it is happening to you, it's very important. And no matter how preliminary our data, heavy drinking is not worth the risks it carries with it, not only in terms of some types of cancer, but obviously its role in liver ailments and other diseases, not to mention the staggering calorie content (approximately 100) of each jigger (1½ ounces) of liquor.

But on the other hand, the overall cancer risk from alcohol must be put in some perspective.

In 1976 about 202,000 American males died of cancer. Some 92 percent of these cancers occurred in sites which have no apparent link with alcohol. That leaves 17,000 deaths. If half of these were caused by alcohol, and that is certainly a very high estimate, that would mean 8,500 cancer deaths were caused by alcoholic drink, 3 percent of all cancer deaths that year. Lung cancer alone, that is, not counting other cancer sites, heart disease or emphysema, accounted for 22 percent of all male cancer deaths that year.

ANY WAY YOU MIX IT, ALCOHOL IS ALCOHOL

In recent years in the United States, there has been a "swing to lightness" in choosing alcoholic beverages. White wine and mixtures of tequila and orange juice (the basis for a Tequila Sunrise) have begun to replace some of the more traditional drinks such as a martini or manhattan. In speaking about alcohol as a possible agent in causing or promoting cancer (and when you consider its general effect on health) it is important to avoid getting caught up in rumors about different types of alcohol having different effects.

For years the rumor around France has been that the red wine produced and drunk in northern France is the cause of cirrhosis—in contrast, wines from other regions and white wines in general are widely considered to be safe for consumption in any amounts. In Spain, cirrhosis has been traditionally associated with port wine—but not with sherry. Germans have long bragged that their good "liver health" was the result of the fact that they drank beer which was free from the devastating health effects of European wines.

At the base of these rumors—and the one that now is leading many Americans to have three glasses of wine instead of one martini—is the belief that whatever ill effects alcohol may have are the result of the concentration of the liquor or the various nonalcoholic components that may be included in it, as opposed to the quantity in the drink itself.

Scientific research provides no basis for such a conclusion. Ethyl alcohol, or ethanol (chemically, CH_3CH_2OH), that liquid with seemingly magical properties and the ability to induce euphoria, sedation, and intoxication, is the same chemical compound no matter how it is served up. Investigations of the physical effects of alcohol ingestion confirm that it makes no difference if you are drinking wine, beer, liqueurs, or distilled spirits. It is the *quantity* of alcohol consumed which is critical.

The comparison of martinis, wine, and beer in terms of alcohol content may seem a bit elusive at first, but the translation of their alcoholic content to a standard base is really very simple. The alcohol content of distilled spirits like gin, whiskey, bourbon, scotch, and vodka, is expressed in terms of the proof. In the United States the proof represents twice the alcohol concentration by volume. Thus whiskey labeled "100 proof" is 50 percent alcohol, that labeled "80 proof" is 40 percent alcohol.

Table wines, carbonated or still, contain about 12 percent alcohol. Although there may be considerable variation in the final product, based on the type of grape used, soil and climatic conditions, harvesting and processing procedures, there is no evidence to suggest that the alcoholic content or physiological impacts of red or white wines are different. Red wines are fermented from red grapes in the presence of the skin; white wines are fermented in the absence of pigmented skin. Consequently, red wines are richer in pigmented compounds and tannin than white wines and contain more acids, potassium, esters, riboflavin, pyridoxine, and nicotinic acids, and less sugar acetaldehyde, thiamine, and, generally, sulphur dioxide, than white wines. But the alcohol content of table wines of any color is relatively constant at about 12 percent.

Fortified wines, on the other hand, usually have a concentration of 20 percent alcohol by volume, the added alcohol consisting of neutral spirits usually made from wine or brandy. Liqueurs range from 20 to 55 percent in alcohol content. And beers, although of different color, aroma, and flavor, are all made by fermenting carbohydrate extracted from barley malt (or rice or corn) and contain 3 to 6 percent alcohol (lager beer) or 4 to 8 percent (stout).

The comparison of three glasses (assuming 5 ounces a glass) of white wine to one martini (assuming it is 3 ounces with a 7:1 ratio of gin to vermouth) is straightforward: 15 ounces of wine x 12% alcohol is 1.8 ounces of pure alcohol; 2.6 ounces of gin x 40% alcohol plus 0.4 ounce of vermouth at 20% alcohol equals 1.1 ounces of pure alcohol. "Never-touch-the-hard-stuff" drinkers can easily consume considerably more booze at lunch than do those who have one traditional drink. Even if one had only *two* 5-ounce glasses of wine, it still would be higher in alcoholic content than the 3-ounce martini (1.1 ounces versus 1.0).

Alcohol, Nutrition, and Cancer

One suggestion on how alcohol may increase cancer risk is based on the possibility that heavy drinkers may not eat a well-balanced diet. If you drink regularly, this is an important factor to keep in mind. Each gram of alcohol metabolized in the body yields seven calories. In terms of everyday calorie counting, that means that 5 ounces of wine adds about 90 or 100 calories, a martini 220, an ounce of 80 proof whiskey or gin 80, and a 12-ounce beer 170.

A nonalcoholic, moderate drinker, then, can quickly accumulate many unnecessary calories and given that alcoholic beverages do not contain significant amounts of protein, vitamins, or minerals, nutrition can easily become borderline. For example, if you have two martinis at lunch, two before dinner and a glass of wine with dinner, you are not only consuming over 5 ounces of pure alcohol—but also nearly 1,000 empty calories. Even if you are following a very liberal daily caloric intake of 3,000 a day, alcohol will account for ⅓ of your total calories. Again, it might be easy to cut back by skimping on food, and "drinking your lunch," even if this involves, for the sake of propriety, ordering a meal and then just not eating very much of it.

Is There a Safe Limit?

Clearly there is a great deal to be learned about the effects of various levels of alcohol consumption on cancer risk. We really do not know at this point how much is too much. Certainly individual susceptibility to alcohol-related problems is a critical factor.

If calories are a source of concern, that reason alone is enough to be moderate about drinking—be it cocktails, beer, or wine. Beyond that, a rule of thumb proposed by a 19th century physician, Francis Edmund Anstie (1833–74), is still widely accepted by those medical specialists who have extensively studied the effects of alcohol. "Anstie's limit," as it is known, states that for a 150-pound man, 1.5 ounces of absolute alcohol per day—3 ounces of whiskey, well diluted; ½ bottle of table wine; or four glasses of beer—taken with meals, will not substantially increase the risk of early death and may indeed, for some individuals, promote both physical, psychological, and social health. Doubling that amount per day, that is, up to the equivalent of 6 ounces of 80 proof liquor, may or may not increase your risk of developing an alcohol-related cancer, or a liver or other type of disorder (but it will certainly have an expanding effect on your waistline). Beyond 6 ounces a day, you may be asking for trouble.

HOW TO PREVENT CANCER

1. As the quotation at the beginning of this chapter suggests, if you do choose to drink each day, turn down the third one. Two per day is enough. Skip the drinks at lunch. Keep your intake of alcoholic beverages below 6 ounces of 80 proof liquor, five 5-ounce glasses of wine, or six glasses of beer.

2. If you do drink every day, try vodka—and keep below the 6-ounce limit.

3. If you must smoke even a few cigarettes a day, *do not make things any worse* by consuming alcohol, even if you are drinking at a time when you're not smoking.

4. If you do drink each day, make sure your alcohol intake does not interfere with your eating a well-balanced meal. In particular, be sure you get enough food with B vitamins and iron, particularly whole grain products, green leafy vegetables, corn, nuts, potatoes, fruits, such as raisins, grapes and peaches, and occasionally, liver.

6

RADIOACTIVITY

"Learn to see in another's calamity the ills
which you should avoid."

Publilius Syrus
c. 42 B.C.

It looked like any ordinary yellow paint. It would blend perfectly
into the standard color spectrum, falling, as all good yellows do,
somewhere midway between red and green. By day it was just
another shade. But by night, it was resplendent, glowing with
seemingly unlimited energy. If you took a magnifying lens to examine its nighttime or darkroom glow, you would see a spontaneous display of miniature fireworks. Diminutive explosions that
blended into brilliance. It was enough to capture the imagination.

In 1915, Dr. Rubin von Hoffmann, a holder of both M.D. and
Ph.D. degrees, thought a great deal about this paint and its potential. He had seen a number of versions of the "magic glowing liquid" and was familiar with the ingredients that yielded the perfect
consistency, tone and, most important, luminescence. He made
his own special version of the paint, mixing a yellowish zinc sul-
phide compound with the essential ingredient for the glow, radium. Experimenting further, he found that a chemical known as
mesothorium, a radioactive isotope of radium and considerably
less expensive, could, when necessary, do the job adequately, either by itself or in combination with radium.

Dr. von Hoffmann in his spare time was an amateur artist. He immediately saw a practical aesthetic application of his paint concoction and noted on one occasion that "pictures painted with radium look like any other picture in the daytime, but at night they illuminate themselves and create an interestingly and weirdly artistic effect." He predicted that this paint would be particularly adaptable for pictures of moonlight or winter scenes and he had "no doubt that some day a fine artist will make a name for himself . . . by painting pictures that will be unique and particularly beautiful at night or in a dark or semidarkened room."

But Dr. von Hoffmann had a sense of business as well as a flair for art. He saw other more economically remunerative uses for his unique radium paint. Specifically, he was familiar with the high-class German and Swiss watches with luminescent dials which derived their glow from mixtures similar to his. A few wealthy Americans had managed to import these specialty items in the previous few years, but because no domestic plant manufactured them, the "night dial" watches were generally unavailable in the States. Recognizing the market and its potential, Dr. von Hoffmann decided to go into the luminescent watch business.

Late in 1915, he and a few associates founded the Radium Luminous Materials Company, and early the following year they established their new company in a two-story factory at the corner of Alden and High Streets in Orange, New Jersey. Soon after moving into their office building, von Hoffmann's group assumed a more corporate-sounding name: henceforth their company was called the United States Radium Corporation.

A staff was quickly assembled. Dr. Edwin Maxon, a twenty-seven-year-old laboratory scientist who had recently received his Ph.D. from the University of Chicago, was appointed chief chemist. Michael Dorland, a forty-eight-year-old laboratory worker with expertise in isolating the precious radium and its isotopes, joined the staff. Von Hoffmann's associates placed an advertisement in the local newspaper announcing that the Corporation was looking for "artists." The ad did not mention that the "art" the group had in mind was painting watch dials. Hundreds of young women—some as young as fourteen, and a few older than twenty-eight—responded and most of them were interested when they learned about the job. Some left high school to take the position. Others had finished their schooling and wanted permanent employment. Still others were only interested in summer or part-time work. The job looked easy. The pay was good. Indeed, the girls were to be paid on a piecework basis and anyone who worked deftly and diligently enough might make as much as one hundred dollars a week. An unskilled worker didn't casually turn down such a promising employment opportunity.

Among the young women who joined the staff of "artists" at the United States Radium Corporation in 1916 and 1917 were Amy Miller, seventeen, and her two sisters, Harriet, nineteen, and Alice, twenty-three. Sally Marton, seventeen, and her sister, Marge, sixteen, Hazel Kelly, fifteen, and Judy Silver, seventeen. Over the next two or three years a few hundred other girls would join them, taking their turns around the large wooden tables in the sun-filled workroom on the second floor (the dial workers referred to it as "the Studio"). Some of the workers stayed for just a month or two, others painted dials for three or more years.

The art of dial painting was a novel one, but relatively easy to learn. The tools of the trade were not complex. Each girl was supplied with a camel-hair brush, a crucible of paint, and a small container of water. The idea was to somehow "tip" the brush so that its point was as sharp as possible, capable of making fine, thin lines on the face of the watch. Accuracy was of utmost importance; sloppily painted watches did not sell. But speed was essential too.

Amy and her two sisters—and many of the other beginners at the Studio—soon found a shortcut which guaranteed improvement in both efficiency and accuracy. If they rolled the brush between their lips before dipping it in the paint, they could easily create that all-important fine point. It was like threading a needle; a quick pull through the mouth flattened out all those messy, loose ends. Sometimes Amy and her coworkers took the time to wash the brush in the jar of water before they "tipped" it; but more often they kept their routine as simple and uncomplicated as possible. They skipped the washing procedure. Tip, dip, dab. Tip, dip, and dab. Of course, in the process of the tipping, dipping, and dabbing, the young women were taking some paint into their mouths. It had a gritty texture and a singularly unpleasant taste. And at the time, the most practical means of getting rid of the disagreeable substance was to swallow it. And swallow it they did. Tipping, swallowing, dipping, and dabbing, each radium-dial painter could finish some two hundred to four hundred watches a day.

Following her sister's pattern, Harriet Miller became particularly efficient at the job. On the average day she would complete at least 350 watches—sometimes more—generally "tipping" her brush through her lips about fourteen or fifteen times per dial. She was fast and accurate and her friends admired, and attempted to simulate, her technique. At least some friends did. Judy Silver, for example, found the whole idea of putting a paintbrush in her mouth very unappealing. She had one or two tastes of the paint and decided she'd do her tipping with water and a cloth, even if it did mean only 200 completed watches per day.

Work as a dial painter was fairly regimented. Usually an austere-looking foreman would stroll up and down the aisles making sure that work on the long tables was moving ahead on schedule. But there were light moments too. The painters used to slip notes into the backs of the watches they knew were going overseas to service men. The watches were cheap ones, and they knew they'd break down fairly soon, and that the young men would look inside to see what went wrong. Sure enough, some eight to ten months after the note was inserted, one of the painters would get a letter from a lonely soldier.

And the glowing paint was a novelty. None of the young women had ever seen anything like it. During the course of the workday, some of the yellow liquid would inevitably be splashed onto their fingers, hands, onto their hair and eyebrows, and certainly on their clothes. When work was done, it was fun to turn the lights out and see who glowed the most that day. It was all very amusing. The painters thought of ingenious ways of using the paint. Some girls would paint their teeth with it before big dates so they would glow romantically when the lights were low. Others would sneak out half-filled vials of the liquid so they could paint their boyfriend's watch in the privacy of their own home. Of course everyone assumed that the paint was harmless. The fact that dust particles from the radium extraction process were all around them didn't bother anyone at all. It didn't deter them from spreading their lunches out at the table at noon, pushing the paint and dust aside as they enjoyed their meal and break.

Indeed, at the time, not very many people knew about the side-effects of this magical physical-chemical substance called radium or about X rays and other radioactive materials.

It was in 1898 that Wilhelm Konrad Röntgen discovered X rays, and just about three years after that, Marie and Pierre Curie were able to isolate that new element they called radium, describing its astonishing ability to give off enormous quantities of energy in a consistent, continuous fashion. People had only good things to say about the new substance. Indeed the Curies and Henri Becquerel, whose work with uranium had prompted their investigations, shared the Nobel Prize in 1903.

It is true that within ten years after the isolation of radium and the experimentation with radioactivity, some medical journals began to report that skin cancer in animals could be induced by excessive exposure to radioactive elements. And in 1914, a French researcher published an account of over one hundred cases of skin cancer among individuals working with these substances. But medical research at that point had not developed to the extent that findings were universally and immediately reported and absorbed by those who might be making decision about how and where radioactive materials would be used. There was certainly no generalized knowledge about any short- or long-term effects from eating the glowing liquid.

Actually, the primary interest in the newly discovered radioactive materials was not in their potential harmful effect, but in their possibilities for use in improving health—specifically for controlling cancerous growths. Radium was tested soon after its discovery as a form of cancer treatment, and the results of early experiments were encouraging.

Unaware of any problems associated with radium, the United States Radium Corporation in East Orange, New Jersey, quickly grew. What started as a company which had contracted with watch manufacturers to paint dials became a major industry which offered the luminescent paint to meet a variety of needs. The dial painters stroked their brushes over light pulls, crucifixes, clocks, and —as the U.S. went to war—painted the faces of a variety of instruments for use on submarines and aircraft. More and more dial painters were recruited. Business was booming. Other dial-painting operations came into existence—in New York, Connecticut, and Chicago. But Dr. von Hoffmann's corporation was the largest and most significant manufacturer of luminescent products.

Then, in the fall of 1922, some six years after the plant had opened, strange things began to happen.

Harriet Miller, one of the first young women to join the team of dial painters, became acutely ill. She had worked at the plant for about two years and then had moved on to another form of work. Around 1920, she developed neuralgialike pains in her legs. Over the course of the next two years, this pain became so severe that she needed a cane to get around. About the same time, Harriet's teeth became loose, her gums bled profusely, and her jaw literally began to disintegrate. She became very weak and was bedridden. On September 12, 1922, she died. She was twenty-five years old.

The Miller family physician was puzzled. The symptoms were indeed bizarre. He filed the necessary papers, registering "ulcerative stomatitis and syphilis" as the cause of death.

Harriet's sisters, Amy and Alice, seemed fine. They were apparently in perfect health. Both sisters had worked at the plant for between eighteen months and two years and had left to be married.

On November 18, 1922, Michael Dorland, age fifty-four, the laboratory worker who had been hired to work with radium, died. He had been a strong, rugged man, weighing some 215 pounds up until a year before his death. His illness overtook him quickly. He simply became weaker and weaker and died. The cause of death was listed as "pernicious anemia."

During late 1922 and early 1923, dentists in the area of the radium plant began to see an increasing number of patients who complained of loose teeth and bleeding gums. Most dentists were puzzled and either recommended pulling all the teeth or suggested that the patient consult medical doctors (who were equally puzzled) for an analysis of the underlying physical cause of the problem. One dental surgeon who was treating a number of women for what he termed "radium jaw" made mention of these isolated cases while addressing a meeting of a dental association. His remarks were published in the *Journal of the American Dental Association*. The notation about radium caught the eye of Harrison S. Martland, M.D., the Chief Medical Examiner of Essex County, New Jersey. He decided to investigate.

By this time, there had been a number of reports in the medical literature about the ill effects of excessive exposure to radioactive materials. Well-known radiologists had died following a period of gradually increasing pallor and anemia. Amputated fingers and limbs, necessitated by the deleterious effects of the radioactive material on skin, were commonly reported by those who worked with X rays. Evidence was mounting that radium was not as harmless as it initially appeared. Maybe the glowing element, which had been ascribed such a bright future, at the time of discovery, had a darker, more sinister side.

In May of 1925, Dr. Martland visited the United States Radium plant. He was appalled at what he found. Individuals entering the area were exposing themselves to an extraordinary amount of radiation. While he was making his report, more tragedies were recorded. Hazel Kelly, one of the youngest and first painters had died. Her symptoms were familiar: her jawbone had deteriorated, she developed acute anemia, became progressively weaker, and finally succumbed to the effects of radium.

In June, 1925, Dr. Edwin Maxon, the company's chief chemist died. Dr. Maxon had noticed his first symptoms just two months before his death, just days after his marriage. He had promised his bride that he would finish his work with radium as quickly as possible and turn to something else. He must have had a suspicion that it was affecting his health, but also felt that his work was so important that it could not be left unfinished. But it was left unfinished. He was thirty-six years old at the time of his death.

That June, Sally Marton also became seriously ill. For the previous three years she had had neuralgialike pains and a severe mouth infection which was diagnosed as pyorrhea. In 1924 she reported to her physician that she bruised easily and was always exhausted. She rapidly became anemic, entered a hospital for treatment, but died on June 26. Sally's sister, Marge, who had worked with the company for six years, was reported at this time to be in critical condition. She died six months later.

Dr. Martland performed an autopsy on the body of Dr. Maxon and found that it contained significant amounts of radium, specifically, twenty-one times the amount considered at that time to be safe. Shortly thereafter, the body of Harriet Miller, the original victim, was exhumed. By this point, Dr. Martland was not surprised to find heavy amounts of radioactive material throughout her body, particularly concentrated in her bones. Harriet Miller *had not* died from "ulcerative stomatitis and syphilis." Indeed she was probably the first human victim of the internal emissions of a radioactive substance.

The problem was clear to Dr. Martland. The radium plant posed a severe health hazard to those entering it. The habit of tipping the paintbrushes between the lips had led to the young women's ingestion of significant amounts of radium and its isotope, mesothorium. Much of the paint a girl swallowed was passed through her gastrointestinal tract and released from her body, but with each "tip" some small, but medically significant amount was added forever to her system. Although the radioactive material would be distributed throughout her entire body, it had a particular predilection for bones.

The answer was equally clear. Don't let anything like this ever happen again. Take precautions when dealing with radioactive materials and, above all, don't eat it. The dangers of radium and its suspected role in the Martland investigation made headlines. And, as expected, the accusations against the miracle element met with opposition. Some of Dr. Martland's associates felt that there wasn't sufficient evidence at that point to make such a judgment. Maybe there was something else "funny" about the New Jersey plant. Their complaints about the bad press radium was receiving was quickly quelled when radium dial painters in other parts of the country died, manifesting the exact same symptoms as did the New Jersey cases. Scientists and laymen alike began to view radioactive substances with a healthy mixture of fear and respect.

One person who had become intensely concerned about the hazards of excessive radium exposure was Dr. von Hoffmann, the company's founder. The evidence convinced him, and he offered his full cooperation in the investigation. One of his most valuable contributions was the work he did on the development of a machine which would measure the extent of radioactive material present in a person's exhaled breath. By using this screening technique, Dr. Martland could identify those who appeared most at risk. When the machine was ready for use, Dr. von Hoffmann offered himself as the first subject. His reading was off the measurement scale. Dr. von Hoffmann was exhaling more radioactivity than any subject they were subsequently to test.

Between 1925 and 1929, Dr. Martland systematically recorded deaths from acute radium poisoning among former dial painters. Some of these young women had left the plant eight or ten years before, but their symptoms were classic and the diagnosis was incontrovertible.

But there were survivors. Not everyone who worked at the radium plant developed the severe anemia and jaw disintegration as did the early victims. For instance, both Amy and Alice Miller, sisters of Harriet who had died from "ulcerative stomatitis and syphilis" in 1922, still felt fairly well, although Amy had developed severe pains in both hips and lower extremities after she had a baby in 1923. Judy Silver, who was among those dial painters who made it a habit not to put the paintbrushes in their mouths, was reported to be in excellent health.

In 1928, the two surviving Miller sisters and three other radium workers, Mrs. Katherine Smith, Mrs. Grace Freeman, and Mrs. Edna Hunt, sued the United States Radium Corporation for damages. The trial was a spectacular one. The headlines in the local papers referred to the complainants as "the five women doomed to die." One concerned man went on radio to plead their case, bringing a set of bones from one of the deceased dial workers. Holding the bones up to the microphone, the listening public could hear the radioactivity they were emitting. "The sound was like peas being dropped slowly into a pan," one listener explained. The press called great attention to the bone broadcast, claiming that dead men (and women) could indeed tell tales.

At the time of the trial, the five girls were in moderately good health. Amy's health, however, had disintegrated some, although she was not developing the classic symptoms that had preceded the death of her sister and other victims.

People around the world had heard of the plight of these young women. Mme. Curie sent her sympathy and advised them to eat raw liver to counteract anemia. A Russian doctor sent a lead solution.

The trial went on for four months. Attorneys for the Radium Corporation maintained that there was a two-year limit on collection of damages for reimbursement for occupational health risks. The attorneys for the women pointed out that the symptoms had not occurred until years after they left the plant. Finally, a judge terminated the case by ordering the Corporation to pay each of the five women $10,000 outright and $600 a year for the rest of their lives—and the cost of all past and future medical services. At the time, such a settlement was considered just and adequate. Not all of those who sued the Corporation were even that lucky. One twenty-seven-year-old former dial painter who was acutely ill from the effects of radium exposure sued the Corporation a number of years after this and was awarded nothing—on the grounds that she had worked as a dial painter at more than one establishment, and no one could be blamed for her current ills.

With the settling of the legal actions against the Radium Corporation in 1928, Dr. Martland thought the bizarre and disastrous incidents were over. The tragedy would thus go down in the history books as one part of the Roaring Twenties that people would not laugh about. There were still many questions that remained unanswered: why did some young women die, and others remain healthy? Well, perhaps there were differences in painting styles; perhaps some dial painters did not "tip" the brush, or did not do so as frequently as others did. And, of course, there remained the possibility that some individuals were more susceptible to the effects of radium than others. Or maybe the survivors used the mesothorium mixture that may not have had the same toxic properties as the radium concoction. But despite the questions, an era of acute radium deaths seemed to have ended.

Then a footnote punctuated what Dr. Martland thought was a final chapter.

Dr. Rubin von Hoffmann, founder of the corporation and mastermind behind the deadly yellow paint, died on November 14, 1928, at age forty-five. In the years prior to his death, Dr. von Hoffmann had lost his front teeth and suffered radium necrosis (tissue degeneration) up to the second knuckle on most of his fingers.

By the mid-1920s, he was acutely aware of the impact radium was having on his health, but he did not hesitate to use it when he thought the conditions called for it. Shortly before his own death, when his sister was suffering from cancer, he personally and extensively treated her with radium in a desperate (although unsuccessful) attempt to save her life.

As is the case with much medical-epidemiological history, it would take more instances of human disaster to prove that this casual approach to radioactive substances was unwarranted.

Dr. Harrison Martland had closed his book on "The Case of the Poisoned Dial Workers" in 1928. With the death of Dr. von Hoffmann, he felt the worst was over and a lesson had been learned at a terrible cost of human lives. But as it turns out, his conclusion was both premature and optimistic. In one sense he was correct: he did not see any more cases of acute radium poisoning. *What he and his medical successors saw over the next thirty years among the radium workers who had painted in New Jersey for some time during the 1917–24 period was cancer.*

On December 7, 1928, Amy Miller, the sister of one of the first victims of acute radium poisoning, died. She was thirty years old. Amy had worked as a dial painter for fifteen months between 1916 and 1917. The cause of death was a "large sarcoma of the right pelvis, infiltrating the bone." Was it possible? Could the substance which was being given so much attention as a possible miraculous cure for cancer actually *cause* this dread disease? Perhaps Amy's death was an aberration. Maybe she would have died at age thirty of a pelvic sarcoma even if she hadn't painted dials.

September 13, 1930. Anna Stacy, thirty-one years old, who had worked as a dial painter for 15 months between 1919 and 1921, died. Cause of death: cancer of the bone.

June 16, 1931. Laura Pearson, thirty, who had worked at The Studio for four years between 1917 and 1921, died. The summer before she had felt a swelling inside her vagina. This gradually became larger and began to interfere with sexual intercourse. When she did finally see her physician, the growth was such that a vaginal examination could not be performed. The malignancy quickly extended; Laura died within a year of her first symptoms.

There was no coincidence here. Carcinomas of any type among women in their twenties and thirties are rare anyway. But three instances within three years among young women who all had been dial painters?

February 19, 1933. Mrs. Katherine Smith, one of the five who had sued the Corporation, died. She was thirty. Katherine had worked as a dial painter for four and a half years, leaving to be married. She slowly lost her teeth, developed excruciating pains in her legs and, for the last few months of her life needed a cane to walk. Cause of death: malignant tumor of the thigh.

October 28, 1933. Mrs. Grace Freeman who had worked painting dials for four years died. She was thirty. Grace was one of the five women who had been awarded $10,000 and an annual pension and medical expenses back in 1928. She was fortunate that medical expenses were included. She had undergone twenty different operations in an effort to restore her deteriorating bones in the years just before her death. Cause of death: carcinoma of the bone.

December 4, 1935. Mrs. Edna Hunt, the fourth of the five women "doomed to die," succumbed to bone cancer. The only surviving member of the group that sued the Radium Corporation was Alice Miller.

Dr. Martland had a partial list of young women who had worked at the Corporation and, as he put it, "with terrible, almost mathematical regularity, I have been crossing off these names," adding to the toll of radium deaths. Reporters used to constantly inquire about what they called "the death list" and Martland would shy away from them. In what had to be one of the all-time understatements, he would reply, "I naturally do not like to talk about it as this list would hardly bring pleasant thoughts to those whose names are on it."

There was a great deal of interest in the cancer deaths of dial painters. *Their deaths provided the first evidence that exposure to radiation could cause internal forms of cancer.* This fact was not established in a laboratory with animals. Many chemicals and physical properties can cause malignancies in rats, mice, and guinea pigs. Vitamin A, for instance, in high doses brings about breast cancer in mice. But the classification of radioactivity as a carcinogenic agent followed this series of human tragedies. The statistics were very convincing, and continued to mount in a manner no one could have predicted.

On November 19, 1946, *thirty years after she had left the radium plant*, Alice Miller, age forty-six, the last of the three painting sisters team, and the last of the five women who had gone to court seeking and receiving payment for damages, died. Cause of death: cancer of the bone.

Helen Gasgo was seventeen when, in 1917, she began to work at the Studio. She painted there for fourteen months, married and had two children, leading a perfectly normal life until 1928 when, more than ten years after leaving the plant, on May 30, while turning to come up from the basement, her right leg snapped. She had fractured her femur. Helen received medical treatment and the bone did eventually heal, although physicians were puzzled about why it took weeks longer than they had expected. On Thanksgiving Day, 1929, after reaching for a platter on a top shelf of her kitchen cabinet, Helen stepped down from the stool and fractured her leg again. This time the bone wouldn't heal. Surgeons tried screws to reunite it. It wouldn't work. Her leg was kept in a cast.

In 1931, Helen Gasgo developed teeth trouble. Her dentist extracted all her teeth. In 1934, her jawbone began to ache, and physicians noted signs of gradual bone deterioration. Through the next twenty years, Mrs. Gasgo's health was only marginal. She had frequent headaches of undetermined origin. By 1955 those headaches became so bad that a prefrontal leukotomy (removal of the white matter in the frontal lobe of the brain) was performed. But in the meantime, she developed a new problem. She had begun to lose her vision in the right eye. By the end of 1955, she was totally blind. In 1956, Mrs. Gasgo lost the ability to move her jaw. It was impossible for her to chew or talk; she had difficulty swallowing, and was admitted to a nursing home. Helen Gasgo died there at age fifty-seven from chronic radium poisoning and carcinoma of the bone. *As a result of fourteen months exposure to radium, forty years before.*

Arthur W. Harmon, who was employed as a chemist at the plant between 1919 and 1922, became the final known statistic in the

New Jersey radium tragedy. He died on August 20, 1960 at the age of seventy-two of cancer of the cheek and jawbone.

Seventy-one occupationally related cancers, fifty-one of them from bone sarcomas, have been identified among 780 dial painters who were painting watches and extracting radioactive material just before, and after, World War I. Incomplete employment records made it difficult or impossible to track down all potentially exposed individuals.

Undoubtedly many more suffered effects and may have died from something else before bone cancer killed them. Only a limited number came to the attention of Dr. Martland (who died in 1954) and his successors. The Atomic Energy Commission in the late 1950s conducted a study, and managed to trace a number of survivors, extracting from them any information they could about former dial workers. One of the women they did find was Judy Silver, one of the original members of the Studio team, who had worked as a painter for two consecutive summers. Judy was in excellent health—describing herself as "fastidious". She explained that at the time she was dial painting, she was the only grandchild her grandparents had—and the only niece of many aunts and uncles. They were very doting, very protective. "Naturally," she told the researchers, "they were not going to let a pretty little girl have anything to do with dirt. And foreign objects were definitely to be kept out of the mouth. Everybody was really quite strict about that—perhaps too strict. I never used lipstick. I never chewed gum. And as a dial painter, I was certainly never going to put a brush that had been swished around in turpentine in my mouth."

Judy's upbringing may have been strict, but there is no doubt about the fact that it saved her life.

RADIUM/RADIATION IN THERAPY

The occupational tragedy involving the radium dial painters was just one in a series of events which led to the dramatic conclusion that exposure to radioactive materials can cause human cancer.

Patent Medicines

During the 1920s and 1930s radium was considered to be a cure-all and got into the hands of "health promoters" like one William J. A. Bailey, who sold the mixture of radium and water as a health tonic. Bailey's product was advertised as being "two hundred fifty times more radioactive than radium" and was guaranteed to solve almost any physical problem, but was particularly recommended for sexual impotence. Radithor came in cases of half-ounce bottles. One bottle was to be taken a day, and it was essential that a patient use the stuff over an extended period for results—a minimum of from three to five years.

Bailey, who frequently assumed the title "doctor," had a great deal of success with his cure-all Radithor, and another of his products "Bioray" which sent off "health promoting" rays derived from radioactive sources. According to "Dr." Bailey, Bioray could "be placed on the desk, by the bed at night, or anywhere else. The rays will pass through the clothing readily so that one can be sure of receiving them even when fully dressed or covered with bed clothing. It is beautifully designed and occupies no more space than an inkwell or desk clock, weighing less than a pound it can be slipped into the handbag to use while one is on a trip. . . . While the Bioray is in the room, it immediately floods it with invisible gamma rays. Thus one can have these rays whenever one desires them. . . . Bioray needs no recharging at any time. The radioactive elements therein will continue to pour a steady stream of rays, day and night, for centuries to come."

Of course Bailey "guaranteed" his products were safe, noting that he himself had consumed cases of the product.[1] He had no reason at that point to suspect he was wrong. On the other hand, he had no good reason to suspect he was right either. But the Food and Drug Administration's power at that point was very limited and individuals like Bailey were free to sell anything they liked. One thing Bailey was right about, however, was the lifetime of the radioactive substance he was selling. It did send off rays for "cen-

1. A check in *The New York Times Obituary Index* shows that William J. A. Bailey died in 1949 of unstated causes. He was sixty-four years old and described as "an inventor and writer." No mention was made of his connection with Radithor.

turies to come." Specifically, it takes 1,622 years for any given bit of radium to lose half its original intensity. Unfortunately, that quality would turn out to be a tragic liability rather than a saleable asset.

When Dr. Martland announced his observations on the effect of ingested radium on the watch-dial painters, Bailey became very defensive. He avidly defended the safety of the substances and maintained that the daily use of his products would ensure the "glow of health." "No one has worked longer or with greater amounts of radium that Mme. Curie," Bailey explained. "For over twenty-five years she has toiled in her laboratory and today is not only much alive, but reported recently to be in excellent health. Someday this famous woman will die either from old age, or some other cause and we will learn that she died 'a victim of radium, a martyr of science.' "[2] Bailey insisted that radium was fine for human consumption and contact, but by the early thirties he voluntarily withdrew Radithor and Bioray because the economic depression made it too expensive for people to buy.

The "Cure" Caused Disease

But throughout the 1930s nonphysicians and physicians alike continued to prescribe radium water as the sovereign treatment for a variety of ills, ranging from gout to skin diseases. Some physicians gave tuberculosis patients radium shots. In 1939, schizophrenic inmates at a hospital in Elgin, Illinois, received regular doses of "radium salts." Their physicians thought this might restore their sanity.

Interestingly, radium may possibly have an immediate beneficial effect on health. The radioactive particles may stimulate the body into defending itself by manufacturing an extraordinary number of red blood cells. These give the victim the illusion of being in excellent health, but the body cannot keep up with such defensive demands for year after year. Eventually disease takes

2. Ironically, these were the exact words that *were* used in the announcement of Mme. Curie's death nine years after this in July, 1934.

over and, in the meantime, radium has been lodged forever in the victims's bones.

The number of people who died from taking patent or prescribed medicines containing radium is even more uncertain than the final death toll among radium workers. Some individuals took bottles of substances while they were in their teens and early twenties and completely forgot about it. Others may have received it from physicians and, unknowingly, ingested radium. For example, one fifty-one-year-old woman complained in 1958 of a painful left knee. Upon examination her physician discovered a malignant tumor which is characteristic of exposure to radium. But this woman had no history of such exposure. She had been a waitress, a file clerk and a saleswoman. And she had never experimented with patent medicines—ever.

Then, shortly before her death she recalled going to a dermatologist in a large city in the Midwest during the 1930s. She had been given weekly injections and a "pink liquid" to be taken by mouth. A follow-up of this lead led investigators to suspect that without her knowledge she had been given a prescription of radium.

During the 1930s and 1940s high dose X rays were used as a treatment for a specific form of arthritis of the spine (ankylosing spondylitis) and to shrink enlarged thymus glands in infants. Follow-up studies showed that deaths from leukemia among these patients was up to ten times greater than in the general population. During the same period, some pregnant women were exposed to diagnostic X rays. Their children demonstrated a twofold excess risk of dying of leukemia before they were ten years old.

Occupational Exposure—Medical

Since radium and X rays were first used, there were scattered reports about how laboratory workers suffered debilitating effects. Loss of fingers, limb amputations to curtail cancer, loss of teeth, hair, blood diseases that weakened the victim, shrunken testes, and decreased fertility. In November 1924, the press gave considerable attention to the death of a Dr. Bergonie, a well-known French radiologist who "was a victim of the weapon he tried to cure others with." Dr. Bergonie had had his right hand amputated and three fingers of his left hand removed. He was suffering from "atrocious pains from the cancerous growths that had invaded his respiratory system." But he was still fascinated with radium. In his last days, he poured radioactive materials on his remaining fingers, watching the results with interest.

Public attention was again called to the dangers of radium when Marie Curie, at age sixty-seven, died of a fatal anemia, most certainly related to her unprotected and continual exposure to the element she and her husband had discovered (Pierre Curie was killed in 1906, run down by a dray in a Paris street). And radium was again in the headlines in 1956 when Marie's scientist daughter, Irene, who had been directly involved with radium since childhood, died of leukemia at age fifty-nine. And again in 1958 when Irene's husband and coinvestigator, Frederic Joliot, died of the same cause at age fifty-eight. In May, 1975, the *New York Times* carried the obituary of Dr. Marguerite Perey, a coworker of the Curies, who succumbed after a fifteen year battle with cancer "believed to have resulted from her work with radioactive materials."

It wasn't until 1944 that the startling incidence of leukemia among radiologists was officially recognized. In each weekly issue of the *Journal of the American Medical Association,* the obituary notes carry the name, medical specialty, age, and cause of death of the members of the association. A casual reader of the *Journal* noticed one day that radiologists seemed to have more than their share of leukemia. A statistical follow-up of his observation confirmed that they had more than three times the incidence of this disease than other physicians. The cause was obvious. Protective measures—both for patients and physicians—became stricter.

Occupational Exposure—Mining

The mines of the Black Forest region of Schneeberg and Joachimsthal in Germany have been worked for their riches for at least the last five hundred years. "Mountain illness" has been recognized for generations. Mountain illness turns out to be lung cancer. It's reported to have affected between 40 and 85 percent of the miners. The problem is that the miners were being exposed to the radioactive effects of uranium. A similar situation has been reported among contemporary uranium miners on the Colorado plateaus.

War

In the years following 1945, more evidence of the cancer-causing effects of radiation became grimly evident. On August 6, 1945, American planes dropped atomic bombs on Hiroshima and Nagasaki. The immediate effects of the bombings were recognized and well publicized: explosions, fires, debris being shot through the air like bullets, human suffering from severe burns, destruction of bone marrow, diarrhea, hair loss. But the *later* effects stemming from one human exposure to an acute blast of radioactivity, are not as well known. Persons who were not killed immediately by the trauma of the blast had *seven to ten times the expected rate of leukemia* (specifically granulocytic leukemia), and significantly increased rates of cancer of the breast, brain, and bowel. Individuals who were under age twenty at the time of the bombing seemed to have been particularly affected. Today, more than thirty years after the atomic blasts, Japanese are still dying from radiation-induced cancers.

RADIOACTIVITY—AND YOU

The human experience with radioactive materials is truly sobering. There is no doubt that any form of ionizing radiation, in sufficient amounts, can induce cancers. The question is, what are we going to do about it?

First, we must acknowledge that although under certain circumstances radiation can be harmful, even deadly, there are circumstances where it has proved invaluable, namely diagnostic X rays, and in the treatment of cancer and other diseases. Second, the degrees of exposure which have led to human death or illness were relatively high. In the case of the therapeutic use of radiation in treating thymic enlargement the dose was about 500 rads. Generally, when you have an X ray at your physician's office, you may be exposed to a tiny fraction of one rad. (It is possible that some of the X ray machines in dentists' offices today emit significantly more radiation than this and possibly should be a source of concern.)

You ought also to be concerned about the radiation threats around you. There are, of course, some sources of radiation that are outside of your control. For instance, what is known as "background" radiation comes from outer space as cosmic rays, some from radioactive elements in the soil, some from isotopes in the air and water. If you live in Denver, Colorado, you are, because of the unusual altitude of that city, exposed to more background radiation than you are in New York City. If you fly in airplanes a great deal you are exposed to more background radiation than if you do not fly often. Of course, one of the most potentially serious for our future, one which is within our control today, is that of man-made sources of ionizing radiation, specifically those associated with atomic testing. One hopes that international maturity and control of nuclear weapons will spare us from increasing the burden of environmental radiation around us.

We simply do not know what role background radiation—or possible leakage from atomic testing—plays or could possibly play in human cancers. The problem is that the evidence we have about the health hazards of radioactive material is based on very large doses, often over prolonged periods of time. We don't know if a few-minute, low-dose exposures over a lifetime add up to pose a threat. Right now the only conclusion we can reach is to proceed with caution, using X rays only when they are a medical necessity. The fact that X ray machines were used during the 1940s and 1950s in shoe stores to ensure good shoe fit, should make all of us shiver.

Mammography

Only thirty years ago, uterine cancer was the leading cancer killer of women in the United States. Since then, the death rate from this disease has declined significantly, the result of a widespread, highly effective means of detection and control. Today breast cancer is the leading cancer killer among American women. With the advent of mammography in the 1960s, there was optimism that breast cancer death rates also could be cut substantially through early detection.

A mammogram is a special X ray of soft tissue that uses lower energy radiation than is ordinarily needed for an X ray image of internal organs. When it was first introduced, the procedure was received with much enthusiasm by both patients and clinicians. But recently some questions have been raised about the procedure, specifically, is the screening method capable of inducing the disease it is supposed to detect? And who should have a mammogram?

In practice, the art of medicine often lies not only in deciding what is beneficial for the patient and what is harmful, but in evaluating which regimen carries the greatest benefit and least risk. This is the central issue in the current controversy concerning the advisability of mammography. The fact that there is a controversy about such a critically needed technique underscores the observation that decisions about the use of known cancer-inducing substances or properties are not easy to make.

In judging the safety of mammography, we begin with the knowledge that exposure to radiation can, and has, caused cancer. The question to be resolved is how much radiation is necessary to have this undesirable effect. In making judgments here, groups such as the National Cancer Institute have reviewed three groups of women, all of whom had been previously exposed to high or very high levels of radiation. These women included the survivors of Hiroshima and Nagasaki atomic bombings, young women irradiated many years ago for postpartum mastitis and another group of young tuberculosis patients who had undergone repeated fluoroscopies. The results of these analyses indicate that while there may be a theoretical risk from low-dose radiation exposure (after a latency period of many years) the risk is extremely small for the individual woman. As pointed out by Dr. Arthur I. Holleb, editor in chief of the journal *Ca—A Cancer Journal for Clinicians,* "Extrapolating from very large doses to very small doses and indicating that there is no absolutely 'safe' dose, it is speculated that if a woman has a mammogram, with approximately one rad absorbed by the breast, her chances of developing breast cancer theoretically change from an expected .07 (7.0 percent) to .0707 (7.07 percent). Stated more simply (if these estimates are applicable here) her probability of eventually developing breast cancer is said to increase from one in 14.3 women to one in 14.1 women."

In making a judgment about the safety of mammography, not only must the possibility of this small, theoretical increased risk of cancer be taken into account, but so must the facts that cancer of the breast is the leading cancer killer among American women and the leading cause of death in women thirty-nine to forty-four years of age. The only recognized approach to saving more lives from breast cancer is detection at a localized, highly curable stage, hopefully before the cancer becomes a mass large enough to palpate. Mammography is the best means available today to screen large groups of women to detect cancer at such an early stage.

Who then should have mammography? Certainly, according to Dr. Holleb and other specialists, all women over the age of fifty should be screened in this manner. For women between the ages of thirty-five and fifty, mammography should be considered for women who are at higher risk of developing breast cancer because they have one or more of the following characteristics:

—chronic cystic mastitis, with or without pain
—lumps and thickenings in the breast
—nipple discharge or other nipple abnormalities
—a personal history of breast cancer
—a family history of breast cancer on the maternal or paternal side
—a family history of breast cancer in sisters
—early onset of menstruation
—no history of pregnancy
—first full-term pregnancy at age thirty or older
—breast surgery scheduled for diagnostic purposes
—fear of breast cancer that requires the reassurance of a negative examination

Clinicians report that some 80 percent of women between thirty-five and fifty years of age will belong to one or another of the above groups that can benefit from mammography. The decision as to which of them should undergo the procedure and how often should be made by the physician and patient.

The unfortunate part of the mammography controversy is that some American women have been frightened into believing that mammography represents only a danger rather than a benefit and a considerable number of women over fifty are now refusing to have the procedure. Any lost opportunity for the early diagnosis of breast cancer with its more favorable prognosis is a legitimate source of concern for everyone involved.

HOW TO PREVENT CANCER

1. Be an alert medical consumer. Choose your physician and dentist carefully. In making decisions about exposing yourself to X rays, you've ultimately got to accept his or her opinion.

2. Keep a record of X rays you've had to avoid unnecessary repetition of exposure.

3. Before you have a dental X ray, make sure you are provided with an X ray protection apron. Because the conditions are not always as controlled in a dental office as they are in a hospital setting, it is possible that the rays are scattered once released, potentially affecting parts other than your teeth. Beware of dental facilities which use X ray machines which are obviously twenty or thirty years old. These machines may emit larger than desirable amounts of radiation.

4. Ask your dentist if he uses "bite wing" or whole-jaw X rays. In the opinion of a growing number of radiologists, the whole-jaw exposure is unnecessary for most dental purposes. If your dentist is going to subject you to a whole-jaw X ray, make sure that there is a legitimate reason.

5. Suggest to your dentist that if it coincides with his medical opinion of your situation, that you would prefer to have your teeth X rayed once, not twice, a year.

6. Do not request diagnostic tests such as mammography just because you hear "everyone is doing it." Mammography is a very useful tool in catching breast cancer in its early stages, but as men-

tioned, because it may carry some small risk it is not routinely used in women under the age of fifty.

7. Unless there is some emergency, do not submit to any type of X ray, dental or medical, if there is any possibility that you are pregnant, even twenty-four hours pregnant.

8. Some medical X rays in the course of a checkup are essential, and the benefits far outweigh the possible risks. For example, smokers over age forty should have a chest X ray *at least* twice a year. Again, mammography for women over age fifty (or other high risk women) is considered by most diagnosticians to be an efficient means of detecting breast carcinomas, a technique where the benefits far outweigh the risks. If your physician is proposing what you feel is an excessive amount of X rays, ask him to explain his rationale. If you still have serious misgivings, seek a second medical opinion.

7

SUN

"Kid, if you had skin cancer, you'd grow a beard too."

Ernest Hemingway

Until relatively recently, fair skin was considered a prize. Queen Marie Antoinette's complexion was described as "an appealing blend of lilies and roses." Some 17th and 18th century French women are reported to have applied leeches to their faces to reduce the superficial blood supply. In Georgian England, ladies painted themselves with material containing white lead. The ability to enchant was based on a dazzling whiteness.

For both men and women, a tanned, weather-beaten complexion has traditionally been regarded as a stigma of the lower classes, pale skin being the trademark of aristocracy. There are people alive today who can recall when a sunbonnet, a picture hat, or parasol was part of almost every woman's wardrobe. The "lady fair" stayed that way because she shunned the sun.

Although some ancients like Herodotus and Hippocrates wrote of the glories of the sun and the Egyptians worshipped sun gods, among whom Ra was preeminent, the use of the sun was primarily limited to religious or specific therapeutic purposes. Prior to this century, examples of white-skinned people voluntarily exposing themselves for prolonged periods to the intense ultraviolet rays of the sun were extremely rare. And so was the incidence of skin cancer.

In 1896. Dr. Paul Unna described a disease which he called "seemanshaut" since it was particularly common in sailors.

Within the next ten years, a number of other researchers reported cases of what they called "tropical skin" among vineyard workers and other outdoor laborers. In 1920, Dr. James McCoy wrote in the *Archives of Dermatology and Syphilology,* "The face, neck and hands comprise but a small surface of the body, yet according to my personal observations 49.6 percent of all cancers are cutaneous cancers of these parts."

But these reports were not of general interest, again because most Americans did not make a habit of broiling themselves in the sun. Both men and women wore sleeved, full-length clothing, and hats, which protected them from the sun's rays. When they did go to the beach, they wore rather elaborate costumes and sat in protected areas.

Things began to change in the mid-1930s. Clothing became lighter. Women became more adventurous about "showing skin." Leisure time increased, and vacations at the beach or in the country became popular. Quite suddenly, "tan" was beautiful. By 1940, both men and women were spending their summer days soaking up the rays, sometimes even inviting a rapid burn by coating themselves with oils, or using a reflector. Some wealthy individuals ensured that they had the "benefit" of a golden tan all year round by going south for the winter.

By the mid-1950s, dermatologists were dealing with an epidemic of skin cancer. Today, this formerly rare disease is the most commonly diagnosed of all cancers in this country.

THE MOST UNIVERSAL CARCINOGEN

There is a great deal of evidence which implicates ultraviolet rays as the prime cause of skin cancer: those with pigmented skin have far less skin cancer than do white people; more than 90 percent of skin cancer occurs on body areas unprotected by clothing—the face, ears, neck, lower lip and back of the hands; skin cancer is much more common in tropical and subtropical areas than it is where the sun is not intense on a year-round basis (on an island just off Panama, the sun causes skin cancer by age six in a significant proportion of the population); fishermen, farmers, professional athletes, and others who work outside are more likely to develop this disease than are those who remain indoors; frequent exposure to ultraviolet rays will induce skin cancer in laboratory animals.

Your skin is multilayered, consisting of the epidermis, the outer layer; the dermis; and subcutaneous layers. But these three are subdivided too. The outer layer of the epidermis, the keratin layer, contains a substance known as melanin (from *melan*, Greek for "black"), a material so dense and insoluble that one scientist who boiled it all night in hydrochloric acid found it unchanged in the morning. It is so durable that it persists in the skin of mummies. When there is enough melanin present in skin, it prevents ultraviolet rays from the sun from damaging the underlying structures. Negroes have a great deal of melanin. Albinos have none.

When you expose your skin to the sun, the immediate result is a slight tan caused by the darkening of whatever melanin is already present. If you have only a slight amount of melanin in your skin, that is if you are fair-skinned, and expose yourself to the sun for only a small amount of time, the melanin you do have will respond and protect you. If your melanin is distributed unevenly, you'll get freckles. Whatever your skin tone, if you get more sun than your skin can handle, a number of skin cells die at once, allowing the ultraviolet rays to penetrate the deeper layers, resulting in tissue change and handicapping the growth of nearby cells. The cellular changes may be very subtle, but if they occur often enough, they apparently set the stage for the development of malignant skin tumors late in life. If you continue to broil yourself in the sun, particularly if you have a fair complexion, you are inviting skin cancer in the same way a cigarette smoker invites lung cancer.

Obviously this does not mean that you should avoid the sun completely. Indeed that would be virtually impossible unless you locked yourself in a dark closet. Even the dermatologists who offer the grimmest warnings on the sun's potential dangers concede that there are circumstances where exposure to its rays can be helpful. The summer sun often relieves asthma, aching joints, psoriasis, and acne. And for most of us a day on the beach can be a relaxing and enjoyable experience. The key here is obviously moderation. The sun's ray's are carcinogenic, but we can use them safely.

AMERICANS AND SUN WORSHIP

If you asked one hundred average Americans, "What causes skin cancer?" probably about 90 percent would say, "The sun." It's fairly common knowledge. That's why it's so puzzling to go to the beach on a sunny July afternoon and see body after body lying there, sometimes for hours, in an intensely hot sun. Perhaps Americans take this particular cancer threat lightly because they feel they derive so much pleasure from the results of sunbathing. They feel healthy and take on what they think is an attractive "outdoors-person" look. Or perhaps they have convinced themselves, consciously or unconsciously, that skin cancer is not a terribly serious disease.

While it is true that 95 percent of skin-cancer patients can become free of the disease if they are diagnosed early and follow a medically approved treatment, the realities are that the surgery for skin cancer can leave unsightly scars and, if the cancer is not found in time, it has the potential for extending to the underlying bone. Skin cancer is cancer and should be acknowledged as such.

But still Americans, as part of their summer ritual, rush to the beach and sit, or lie, unprotected in the sun. One can't help but think of the lemmings who bring on their own doom with the fatal stampede into the sea. The honey-blonde young woman who is in a bikini lying gloriously on the beach towel, shimmering with baby oil, is either unaware, or chooses to overlook the fact, that by doing so she is ensuring that by the time she is thirty, her skin will look like age forty, and her odds on developing skin cancer by age fifty will be remarkably high.

Teen-age girls seem to be the most difficult group to convince about the dangers of the sun. The "tan is beautiful" fashion has caught their attention and somehow age fifty-five seems a long way off. Tragically, most dermatologists now believe that it is the exposure to excessive amounts of intense sunlight during the teen years which initiates the carcinogenic process in the skin's tissues. Of course, continued exposure during the twenties, thirties, and later makes the situation even worse. But the skin is most sensitive among individuals under age twenty.

PROTECT YOURSELF FROM THE SUN!

The hazards posed by excessive exposure to sunlight have been well known to dermatologists for decades. Unfortunately, the concern is not generally shared by the public and throughout this century there has been a growing fascination with sun worship, literally basking in the intense sunlight, inviting the many problems which go with abuse of the sun's warming rays: premature aging of the skin, loss of skin elasticity, skin dryness, leatherlike skin, and most serious, skin cancers.

Just about everyone—but particularly those with fair complexions—is familiar with the discomfort of sunburn: the redness, swelling, and tenderness, perhaps accompanied by nausea, dizziness, and weakness, that results from getting too much sun too fast. And at some point, almost everyone has tried a "suntan lotion" either to accelerate tanning or to offer some protection from the burning rays. Understandably, however, if you enter a drugstore in search of such a product, you may be confused by the variety of materials available to you.

Choose your sunscreen or sun-tanning preparations carefully. Not all are equally effective. Baby oil, mineral oil, and olive oils do *not* protect skin from sunburn—indeed, they may invite a painful burn by intensifying the effects of the rays. They are *not* recommended if you are interested in keeping your skin healthy and young-looking.

You may be offered various products which promise to tan you without sun. Most of these contain a product known as DHA (dihydroxyacetone) which when rubbed into the skin combines with free amines to produce a brown coloration in about two to five hours. This effect is not very long lasting. It begins to disappear after about two or three days and is completely gone in about a week. And many observers are quick to notice that you have a "tan from a bottle" because of the evenness of the color, if not because of the suddenness of its appearance. But the main problem with such preparations is that they may lead you to asume that the artificial tan confers the same type of sun protection as would a tan from the sun's rays. This is not necessarily so—unless the preparation has a screening agent—and you may be asking for a painful sunburn if you go basking with your artificial tan.

Sunscreens, of which there are two types, offer the most practical and efficient means of avoiding the harmful rays of the sun. Physical sunscreens are just what the name implies: they provide a barrier to sunlight. Clothing, hats, umbrellas, or in days past, parasols, serve such a function. Additionally, liquid preparations such as oxide of zinc, which in effect offer you a liquid mask to place on your skin, will serve as a physical sunscreen.

Chemical sunscreens offer another form of protection, the idea being that a sun-screening lotion will absorb the light of a particular wavelength, allowing you to sit in direct sunlight, but filtering out the harmful rays. With a sunscreen you can achieve a slow, even tan, without insulting your sensitive skin tissues.

There are a number of sun-screening products available in your local drugstore, but again, some are more effective than others. Those containing PABA (an abbreviation for the chemical para-aminobenzoic acid) are generally considered the most desirable (PABA solutions are sold under a number of brand names, including PreSun and Pabanol). These lotions do have the disadvantage of causing allergic reactions (contact dermatitis) in a very small number of people—and occasionally they can leave a permanent yellow stain on the clothing. Another category of screens containing esters of PABA (sold under names such as Block Out, Eclipse, Pabafilm and Sea and Ski) offer relatively good protection, although not as good as the PABA solutions themselves, and do not stain clothing.

No sunscreen is completely effective. First, no matter what type you choose, you should apply it frequently. Needless to say, the lotion will wash away or become diluted after swimming or after sweating for many hours on a hot beach. Second, even with a sunscreen, it is not recommended that you broil yourself for hours in the sun. Moderation is still the key.

So if you are headed for the beach—or the country, or the ski slopes—choose an effective sunscreen and use it frequently and liberally. Don't be fooled by cloudy days. The rays can still get through to your skin and you need the screen if you are sitting out for a long period of time in an unprotected area.

HOW TO PREVENT CANCER

1. Don't broil yourself in the sun. This is particularly important for fair-haired, blue-eyed individuals, but common sense about sun exposure applies to everyone.

2. When you are sitting in direct summer sunlight for more than fifteen minutes, use a sunscreen which contains PABA.

3. Once you've applied the lotion, start your sunbathing with fifteen minutes of exposure, adding on five-minute increments each day.

4. Minimize your exposure to direct summer sunlight between the hours of 11 A.M. and 2 P.M.

5. Beware of cloudy days. Invisible ultraviolet radiation can penetrate almost anything. On those days "scatter" caused by drops of moisture suspended in the overcast allow 80 percent or more of the normal ultraviolet tradition to come through. Ireland, known for its cloudy weather, has nearly as high a skin cancer rate as does sunny Australia.

6. Remember, while umbrellas at the beach are some help in protecting you from the sun, they block out only 55 to 60 percent of the ultraviolet rays. The rest are reflected onto you and from the sand and water.

7. Be particularly cautious of the sun in tropical countries, at high altitudes. Every thousand feet above sea level carries a 5 percent heavier ultraviolet penalty.

8. Take sun precautions when you ski. Snow reflects about 80 percent of ultraviolet rays.

9. Do not use baby oil, coconut oil, or related materials to promote tanning. Do not use a reflector.

10. When you go to the beach, bring some light-colored, long-sleeved, tight-weave clothing and use it to protect yourself. If you are prone to sunburn, bring a hat too—and wear it.

8

DRUGS

"There are remedies worse than the disease."

Publilius Syrus,
c. 42 B.C.

In the late-1940s, Susan and Jim Peterson, and their five-year-old son, Tommy, moved to a suburb of Boston, Massachusetts. The Petersons had always planned on having a large family—five children at least. They were both from large families themselves and enjoyed home life and family activities.

But things did not work out the way they planned. They were married for ten years before their first child was born. Prior to his birth, Susan had experienced four miscarriages. When Tommy was born they were overjoyed and eager to seek another pregnancy as soon as possible.

When in January of 1949 Susan became pregnant again, her obstetrician, a suburban doctor with a part-time teaching appointment at the Harvard Medical School, decided to take no chances. There was a new drug—stilbestrol—which apparently worked wonders with cases where miscarriage was threatened. Given Susan's age (she was now thirty-six) and history of pregnancy loss, he felt stilbestrol was definitely indicated. She started on the tablets immediately after her pregnancy was confirmed, and gradually increased the dosage until just prior to the delivery date.

In October of 1949, Susan gave birth to Anna an eight-pound six-ounce, healthy baby girl.

Anna's growth and development during childhood was uneventful. She was just like any other girl, having her share of good health and illness. She did distinguish herself in two ways: First, she was an honors student at the private school she attended in Connecticut. Second, she was an outstanding athlete, her favorite sport being swimming.

In June 1970, Anna graduated from high school and that fall entered a prestigious women's college. In late September she began to experience heavy vaginal bleeding between menstrual periods, but she didn't take it too seriously. Many girls found that their periods were thrown off schedule by the excitement of starting college life. The bleeding stopped for a while, but became heavier in November, and even heavier in December. The college physician referred her to a gynecologist in Boston. Anna was examined while she was home for Christmas vacation. During the exam, the gynecologist found some unusual vaginal ridges. Her cervix was an odd strawberry color. A biopsy was taken and the grim results were soon in: Anna had a rare cancer—adenocarcinoma—of the vagina. She was immediately hospitalized and underwent a full hysterectomy and vaginectomy (removal of the vagina).

THE INTRODUCTION OF A "MIRACLE" DRUG

In England in 1938, Dr. E. C. Dodds and his coworker made a discovery which was received with great enthusiasm in the medical world: they had discovered a way of synthesizing a form of estrogen. Until this time estrogens were only available from pregnant mare's urine and other natural sources. They were not only too expensive for general practical use, but were difficult to prepare and highly ineffective when used orally.

The new estrogen, stilbestrol, which was chemically very close to natural estrogen, capable of producing all the physiological effects of the natural hormone, corrected all these difficulties: it was inexpensive, potent and capable of being administered in the form of a pill.

The real excitement about stilbestrol was in the area of treating menopausal symptoms. In a November 1941 issue of *Today's Health* magazine (then known as *Hygenia*), an article entitled "Help for Women over 40" sang the praises of the new drug, noting its effectiveness in relieving pain, discomfort, crying spells, sleeplessness and "nerves." A professional paper published in 1941 in the *Journal of Clinical Endocrinology* raved that "stilbestrol, a new synthetic estrogen, has extraordinary clinical possibilities." In addition to treating menopausal women, stilbestrol was immediately seen as a drug to control prostate cancer.

While stilbestrol use was steadily increasing among older women and men with various symptoms of menopause or disease, other physicians had some expanded ideas for the drug. In May 1943, a doctor writing in *Medical Times* suggested that stilbestrol was not being utilized as much as it should be: "When a drug has become definitely associated with one phase of medicine, it may be overlooked that there are other uses. So it is with stilbestrol." The writer went on to note that while it was "outstanding" in managing menopausal symptoms, it should also be used in pregnancy testing, treatment of nausea of pregnancy, and treatment of threatened or repeated miscarriage.

By 1948 a whole series of medical journals were recommending the use of stilbestrol during pregnancy. In that year, a physician from San Francisco, told the *American Journal of Obstetrics and Gynecology* that "the use of stilbestrol for the prevention or treatment of disease has brought to our specialty one of the most exciting and controversial topics in recent years." In 1950, the two major pharmaceutical companies listed in the *Physician's Desk Reference* recommended large doses of stilbestrol for threatened abortion, specifically advising that women be given 5 mg. in the seventh week of pregnancy, with a stepwise increase to 135 mg. at the thirty-fifth week, then discontinuing it.

Some writers in the late-1940s and 1950s went so far as to suggest that stilbestrol be administered to *all* pregnant women during pregnancy, whether or not they had a history of miscarriage, to prevent or decrease the hazards of late complications of pregnancy for mothers and the babies. Undoubtedly, some American physicians followed this recommendation.

During this time there were scattered reports of some undesirable side effects of stilbestrol ingestion among nonpregnant women. For instance, when some young children accidently received the drug in place of their regular prescription (because of an error in drug manufacture), the three- and four-year-old girls began to have "menstrual periods" and exhibit other symptoms of sexual precocity. When adult men were treated with the drug, it often had a stimulating effect on their breasts, and caused them to lose their sexual drive.

Some physicians thought this latter observation had some practical application and recommended that stilbestrol be given to male sexual criminals to control their urges.

The rumblings about the possible ineffectiveness of stilbestrol in pregnancy began in the early-1950s. Although in 1952 one team of physicians went on record in the *New York State Medical Journal* as stating that "the clinical experience and experimental data published to date appear to establish a sound basis for the use of stilbestrol in many complications of pregnancy," others, like Dr. D. Robinson and Dr. Landrum B. Shettles in the same year were reporting that "in careful comparisons . . . there was no evidence that stilbestrol increased the pregnancy salvage rate."

In 1953 the evidence against the usefulness of stilbestrol in pregnancy became even stronger (there was, however, no mention of any side effects of the drug, certainly not a suspicion of cancer). Gradually, most obstetricians stopped using the drug, but as late as 1970, despite all the medical evidence to the contrary, some United States obstetricians continued to prescribe the drug "to prevent miscarriage."

In 1966, Dr. Howard Ulfelder, a gynecologist at the Vincent Memorial Hospital, the gynecological service of the Massachusetts General Hospital saw a sixteen-year-old girl with unusual vaginal bleeding patterns. He made the diagnosis of adenocarcinoma of the vagina. Cancer of the vagina is rare, occurring usually in women over age fifty. So this case was very puzzling.

Between 1966–70, seven girls, ages fifteen to twenty-two with this same disease were seen at Vincent Memorial Hospital. What was it that these girls could have in common? What could explain their suffering from such a rare disease at such an early age?

Dr. Ulfelder, and his associates Drs. Arthur L. Herbst and David C. Poskanzer, confirmed that the victims did not uniformly use any intravaginal irritant, douches, or tampons. Only one patient had had sexual exposure. Before the onset of their illness, none used birth control pills. By comparing these seven girls to other women the same age who did not have vaginal cancer, they found a highly significant relationship between the occurrence of the disease, and the treatment of the victims' mothers during that pregnancy with stilbestrol. All the mothers who took stilbestrol began therapy in the first three months of pregnancy.

The Boston doctors published their grim findings in an April 1971 issue of the *New England Journal of Medicine*. That report came *thirty years* after stilbestrol was first used as a drug in this country, twenty-eight years after a report in *Medical Times* suggested that the drug be used in pregnancy, twenty-one years after Susan Peterson began taking large doses of it to "prevent miscarriage."

It was the timing of this drug so early in the gestational period that apparently was responsible for the tragedies. The fetal vaginal cells at that point are very susceptible to hormones, and may have undergone the initial malignant transformation while still in the womb. The hormonal changes of adolescence, fifteen years afterward, restimulated a malignancy that had already begun.

Following the report by Drs. Ulfelder, Herbst, and Poskanzer, other researchers around the country—and around the world— submitted similar results. Registries for reporting this disease were set up, so adequate statistics could be compiled. Research in this area was difficult because many mothers simply could not remember whether or not they took medication during pregnancy. But when old medical records were dug out, they almost always confirmed that mothers of daughters with adenocarcinoma of the vagina took "hormones" during pregnancy, generally very early in the pregnancy.

How Many Women at Risk?

It has been estimated that between 100,000 and 160,000 females born in the United States between 1960 and 1971 were products of pregnancies in which the mothers were given stilbestrol. No estimates of the number of women given the drug between 1947 and 1960 are available, but the number is probably much more than 160,000. Presumably, hundreds of thousands or millions of girls were exposed.

As of 1974, after a thorough nationwide medical search, only about one hundred cases of stilbestrol-associated cancers have been uncovered. Thus, it is likely that the risk of cancer development following exposure to this drug is considerably less than four in one thousand. If diagnosed early, adenocarcinoma is curable, usually through major surgery. In the cases where the vagina has been removed, there have been successful building of artificial vaginas which allow normal sexual intercourse. Obviously, given the hysterectomy which is generally necessary, childbearing is not possible.

In addition to the cases of vaginal cancer, a small group of women whose mothers received stilbestrol during pregnancy develop vaginal or cervical adenosis, unusual glandular cells in the vagina. Adenosis may be a premalignant change, that is, a stage which if not given prompt medical attention, could become cancerous. Adenosis is usually treated locally, often using progesterone suppositories which oppose the effects of natural estrogens and generally lead to a disappearance of the problem.

It is clear from these figures that an extremely small percentage of exposed women manifest any form of vaginal or cervical disease. But because of the seriousness of the syndrome, all women who suspect that they may have been exposed prenatally to stilbestrol should bring this to the attention of their gynecologist at every yearly, or preferably, semiannual, vaginal examination.

Are the Sons of Stilbestrol-Treated Women at Risk?

Some very preliminary evidence suggests that a small portion of sons of these treated women might have an increased incidence of reproductive tract abnormalities such as cysts and small testicles, and possibly a higher than normal frequency of infertility. There have been no reports of increased cancer risks in males who were prenatally exposed to stilbestrol.

MEDICINE AND CANCER: RISKS AND BENEFITS

The stilbestrol incident is one of many cases where it was learned, after the fact, that a drug increased the patients' probabilities of developing cancer. It was the first known instance of what is known as "transplacental carcinogenesis."

In some cases, looking at them in retrospect, the cancer-causing potential of the drug was unacceptable given its purpose—and as a result those drugs or forms of treatment are no longer being used. For instance, the use of high doses of radioactivity as the "cure" for an enlarged thymus in childhood, and the subsequent increase in leukemia, was considered one of the low points in the history of medical therapy. Other low points included the use of *thorotrast*, a radioactive substance used around the world between 1930 and 1950 as a contrast medium for diagnostic purposes, which led to liver cancer in a significant number of the patients who received it; *chlornaphazine* (which might have been suspected of being carcinogenic in that it is a derivative of beta-naphthylamine, the industrial carcinogen) after it caused bladder tumors in patients with Hodgkin's and other diseases who were being treated with it; and *inorganic arsenic* compounds, formerly used in dermatology as "Fowler's solution," because they cause human skin cancer.

But still other drugs with the capability for increasing the risk of cancer are still considered acceptable because the benefits outweigh the possible risks. For example, immunosuppressive agents, which are absolutely necessary in minimizing the chances of rejection of kidney transplant recipients, are suspected of increasing the patient's risk of developing a number of types of cancer. Apparently, when the immunosuppressive drugs become effective, they turn off much of the body's "surveillance system," leaving the patient vulnerable to cancer. Certain drugs which are used in cancer therapy may pose human cancer risks—but in many cases they have proved useful and the risks are considered in these circumstances to be acceptable.

Under Investigation
AMPHETAMINES

Amphetamines, taken mainly for weight reduction, recently have been linked with a sixfold risk of Hodgkin's disease. While these charges against the drugs are under investigation, it would seem wise to minimize our exposure to amphetamines.

RESERPINE

A drug used in treating hypertension, reserpine may increase the patient's likelihood of developing cancer of the breast. This new lead is also being intensely evaluated.

ORAL CONTRACEPTIVES

While there is no significantly increased cancer risk in women who have used The Pill for a number of years—and indeed the medication may offer some slight protection in the case of breast cancer, it is still being studied. Given the long latency period of cancer, there is some cause for concern. Oral contraceptives have only been available since 1960 and in widespread use since 1965. A great many women who have taken the drug now for twelve or more years did not begin taking it until they were over age twenty-five or thirty. We still have much to learn about the effect of the oral contraceptive when therapy is begun early, say at age sixteen, and continued for thirty or more years.

POSTMENOPAUSAL ESTROGENS

In the past three years, there has been much discussion about the possible cancer-inducing effect of postmenopausal estrogens like Premarin, a drug used in treating uncomfortable menopausal symptoms like hot flashes, palpitations, vaginal dryness.

Two studies recently reported that women taking estrogen have a five to fourteen times as high rate of endometrial cancer (that is, cancer of the lining of the body of the uterus) than do women of the same age not taking the drug.

This increase should be put in perspective: an obese woman, simply because of her weight, is increasing her chances of developing uterine cancer by three- to ninefold. A smoker increase his risk of developing lung cancer by as much as ten- to seventeenfold.

As of this writing, the verdicts on these drugs are not in yet, but the general message is "proceed with caution," using the lowest dose levels possible.

COULD WE PREVENT DRUG TRAGEDIES?

Couldn't animal studies predict in advance that a drug could cause human cancer? Not necessarily. Some drugs are carcinogens in animals, but apparently not in man. For instance, isoniazid, used in the control of tuberculosis, induces lung adenomas in mice, but not in rats or hamsters. Sodium penicillin when injected into rats causes sarcomas, but from what we know of its use in humans, it is not a cancer risk. The female steroidal hormones used in the oral contraceptives have been known for years to cause cancer in laboratory animals.

If we were to make judgments on the basis of the rat alone, The Pill would never have been introduced.

In many cases, the drug-induced cancer deaths were not predictable and in that sense were not preventable.

But in the case of the drug stilbestrol, there was obviously gross negligence on the part of physicians who continued to administer the drug during the 1960s—and even as late as 1970—when it was clear that there was no purpose for it (that is, it did not decrease miscarriage risk) and evidence on the carcinogenic potential of all hormones in large doses was mounting quickly. All that can be said is that medical communication was still not fully developed during those years, and practicing physicians who did not keep up with the literature were simply not informed.

The history of drug-induced cancers does make us look at this area with great caution. Unlike the case of food additives (which we'll turn to in Part II) drugs are not used by humans in trace amounts, but rather at relatively high dose levels.

In evaluating drugs it is sobering to realize that our animal testing can only provide us with warnings. They cannot predict effects in another species with absolute certainty. Decisions must be made on the basis of a number of observations, the extent to which the drug causes malignancies in animals (Is it just one species and one organ affected or does the drug induce carcinomas in many different animals at many diffrent sites?), the purpose of the drug and the alternatives which may be available, the chemical structure of the drug (Is it chemically similar to any known carcinogens?), and ultimately, on the basis of clinical drug trials involving human beings.

HOW TO PREVENT CANCER

1. Never, under any conditions, take any drug, even an over-the-counter one, during pregnancy without first checking with your physician.

2. Reduce your consumption of all drugs, over-the-counter as well as prescription.

3. If you are using the oral contraceptive, reevaluate occasionally that decision to ensure that you are deriving sufficient unique benefits from it to warrant whatever risks may be involved. At this point there is *no* convincing evidence that the oral contraceptive increases cancer risk. But the frightening aspect here is that the same thing could have been said about stilbestrol use in pregnancy in 1970, almost thirty years after it was first introduced.

Unlike other forms of medication, the oral contraceptive is generally "patient prescribed" for a purpose (pregnancy prevention) which in some, although not all circumstances, can be accomplished by nonhormonal means.

4. Choose your physician carefully. In accepting drugs, you must ultimately base your decision on his opinion. If practical, choose a physician who has some type of medical school or other university affiliation. He may be more likely to keep up to date with medical events and possible adverse drug effects.

5. If you have reservations about one physician's opinion on a controversial drug (like Premarin, reserpine), do not hesitate to get a second medical opinion.

6. If you are a woman who has reason to believe that you were prenatally exposed to stilbestrol, call this fact to the attention of your gynecologist. Have pelvic examinations at least twice a year. Precancerous lesions can be detected and dealt with.

9

SEX

> "Tumors of this sort [of the breast] are found
> more often in nuns than in any other women.
> In my opinion, these tumors [are due] to the
> celibate life led by these women."
>
> Bernardino Ramazzini, 1700

Does sex cause cancer too? Is there not any pleasurable aspect of life that does not carry a cancer risk?

Evidence gathered over four centuries clearly points to the fact that certain patterns of sexual and reproductive behavior can increase your risks of developing cancer of the cervix, uterus, and breast. To a lesser extent, sexual patterns may also affect odds on cancer of the penis and prostate gland. Some of the associations made between reproductive and sexual factors have some practical application, if not for you, for your children or grandchildren. Others, however, simply do not have a practical application because they are based on biological aspects of our lives over which we have little or no control.

CANCER OF THE CERVIX

In 1905 a New York City gynecologist, Dr. H. N. Vineberg, discovered that one of his patients had cervical cancer. What surprised him was not finding a case of this form of cancer—he had seen it before—but the fact that the woman was Jewish. In Vineberg's experience, this disease rarely affected Jewish women. As a result of this observation, he did considerable research in his files and noted that cervical cancer was far more common among his non-Jewish patients—twenty times more frequent than among Jews. Dr. Vineberg's statistics are just one of many which have contributed to our knowledge about the causation of cervical cancer.

Women who begin having sexual intercourse early in life, that is, before age eighteen, have two to three times the frequency of cervical cancer as do women who experience their first coitus at a later age. Women who have both early sexual experience *and* multiple sexual partners during their lifetime are at an even higher risk of developing this disease.

Imprisoned prostitutes have a four- to sevenfold higher rate of cervical cancer as compared with other female inmates.

In the United States, nonwhite women have two and a half times the mortality from this disease as compared to white women.

For many years it was assumed that the increased cervical risk that some women have was the result of their having many children, rather than the sexual exposure itself. But this explanation is no longer accepted. Indeed, much of what we know about this malignancy suggests that it is a type of venereal disease, one to which young women are particularly vulnerable. Women who begin having intercourse early are apparently most at risk because their adolescent cervical tissues are in the state of flux at that time and particularly sensitive to whatever the sexually transmitted cancer-causing or pre-cancer-causing agent. Although the disease may not become evident until she is forty or fifty years old, the carcinogenic process may be initiated in the teens.

What Causes It?

Perhaps, it has been suggested, the risk of cancer of the cervix is enhanced by poor male hygiene, specifically, an accumulation of smegma, the thick cheesy secretion under the prepuce of the penis. This might account for the low risk of women married to Jewish men, all of whom are, as dictated by religious dogma, circumcised. Circumcision makes genital hygiene easier, preventing smegma accumulation.

A multitude of experiments have attempted to find a carcinogen in smegma—painting it on animals, injecting it into them. But no tumors could be induced.

Or perhaps there is a carcinogen in semen itself. The male ejaculate is made up of hundreds, if not thousands, of chemicals. It would be difficult to identify which might be involved. But if there is a base to the belief that the semen or some portion of it is a causative agent, those using a condom or diaphragm might be expected to have lower rates of cervical cancer, even though they did become sexually active at an early age. But this type of study is yet to be done.

Some interesting research which suggests that cervical cancer may somehow be transmitted from male to female is being conducted by Dr. Irving Kessler, a professor of epidemiology at Johns Hopkins. Dr. Kessler has noted in preliminary results that women married to widowers whose previous wives had died from cervical cancer have four times the frequency of this disease as compared to a closely matched group of women in a control population. For him, this implies that some men are capable of passing on the risk of cervical cancer to certain susceptible females.

Herpes Virus II

Over the past ten years, there has been increasing evidence that herpes virus "type 2" may be a causative agent in the development of cervical cancer.

Herpes is the medical designation for a condition more commonly known as a "cold sore" or "fever blister." In recent years it has been determined that there are two types of viruses in this category: "type 1," those blister-type infections which occur in the areas of the mouth and face, and "type 2," which generally affects the genital organs.

Herpes genitalis, or "type 2" is now occurring with increasing frequency in both sexes and there is abundant evidence for classifying it as a venereal disease: it predominates in sexually mature people, is often diagnosed in the sex partners of affected patients and is associated with other sexually transmitted diseases, like gonorrhea and syphilis.

The herpes lesions appear on or near the sex organs, some three to seven days after sexual intercourse with an affected person. The sore will take the form of clusters of tiny blisters which may rupture in a day or two to cause shallow ulcers. The disease is usually self-limiting, that is, it clears up without treatment, usually within about six weeks and leaves no scar. But during the course of the disease the patient may complain of burning and pain, fever and a "flulike" illness or tiredness. Additionally, second attacks of herpes genitalis frequently occur over a period of the next few years *without* new venereal contact, precipitated only by emotional or physical trauma, menstruation, or some other event.

The second attack is usually of shorter duration and less severe, but may cause anxiety for the patient merely because of its recurrent nature. There is no specific treatment for either the primary or secondary episodes of herpes genitalis, other than bathing with a weak saline solution to relieve discomfort. As with all forms of sexually transmitted diseases, the primary means of prevention is avoidance of sexual contact with an affected person.

Examinations of women with cervical cancer have revealed a positive association between that disease and the presence of herpes virus "type 2" antibodies. Some recent studies point to a link between animal tumors and herpes virus strains. Thus among women who have early and frequent sexual encounters with a variety of men, the herpes virus may initiate or promote malignancies of the cervix.

A relationship between herpes genitalis and cervical cancer is far from being confirmed and there have been a number of puzzling observations in this area of study (for example, repeated injections of "herpes 2" in the cervix of monkeys does not have any cancerous effect). But in a sexually free society, where attitudes and behavior of young couples has recently shown marked change, the question of an association between cancer of the cervix, early sex in general, and herpes genitalis in particular, obviously merits urgent attention. What is particularly unsettling is that not only are young women having sex earlier, they are using the oral contraceptive, not a local form of contraceptive such as a condom, that might possibly offer some protection.

BREAST CANCER[1]

As Ramazzini stated in the eighteenth century, nuns are more likely than other women to develop breast cancer. Indeed, this is true of all unmarried women. But the explanation for this is not, as Ramazzini stated, the fact they are leading "celibate lives," but rather due to the fact that they have not had children.

Since that time, we've learned more about the association of childbearing and breast cancer. Not only does it make a difference if you have a child or not, but the *age* at the birth of your first child has a part in determining risk. Women whose first baby is born before they are eighteen years old have one-third the risk of those whose first baby is born after age thirty-five. The relationship here applies only to the first birth.

In terms of percentages (so that you can compare this to life's other risks), women becoming mothers for the first time after age thirty-five have a 20 percent greater risk than those who do not have children at all, and a 30 percent greater risk than those who had a baby early in life, of developing the disease. When you compare that to something like the cigarette risk range of 400 percent to 1,000 percent or more, you can see the difference in the nature of the problem.

Breast Feeding

Is it having a child early in life—or is it breast feeding—which offers some protection?

1. The cancer risk factors here generally also apply to the body of the uterus (as opposed to the neck of the uterus, the cervix) and the ovary.

The idea that lactation lowers breast cancer risk has been around for at least fifty years. But, Dr. Brian MacMahon, Dr. Philip Cole, and their associates at the Harvard School of Public Health, who have spent years studying the causation of human breast cancer, have concluded that lactation has little, if any, effect on breast cancer risk. If there is any effect, they state, "It is too small to be demonstrable even in large series of cases."

Cancer of the Breast and Hormones

It has long been thought that certain types of estrogen, natural or artificial, increased the risks of breast cancer. According to this theory women who have children, especially when they have them early, have lower risks of this disease because their body produces progesterone, "the hormone of pregnancy," which opposes estrogen, at least temporarily, giving them a "break" from what otherwise would be a continual exposure to the potentially cancer-causing effects of natural estrogen.

Three specific types of estrogen are under study. Two, estradiol and estrone, regularly produce mammary tumors in rats; the third, estriol, apparently does not. The suggestion is that estriol may "resist" the action of the other two fractions. Perhaps the events of pregnancy influences the ratio of these natural chemicals in a woman's body in a way that reduces the odds on the growth of breast tumors.

Most recently, the research on the hormonal cause of breast cancer has focused on prolactin, a hormone released by the pituitary gland. Women taking a drug known as reserpine, which in some complex way increases the flow of prolactin, apparently have a two- to fourfold risk of breast cancer. Prolactin also increases susceptibility of breast cancer in rodents. Perhaps different women have different natural levels of prolactin. Or maybe dietary factors affect blood prolactin levels (a recent study of a small number of women showed that high fat diets did lead to elevated prolactin levels).

But what is puzzling in the prolactin theory is that the levels of this hormone *rise* during pregnancy. If it does play a role in human breast cancer perhaps women are only sensitive to it at a certain age, say beyond the early- or mid-thirties, or in some special set of biologically and environmentally determined circumstances.

The ultimate answer will probably be that "breast cancer" is actually a variety of different diseases, some hormonally determined by a multitude of internal and external circumstances.

Breast Cancer and Other Factors

The fact that the age at first birth affects a woman's breast cancer risk is of limited practical use. If a woman who believes in the traditional means of family formation, doesn't get married until she is thirty-two, she does not have the option of having a child at an early age.

Some other information we have about increased cancer risks has even less practical application and thus will only be mentioned here in passing. Women who begin menstruating early in life, that is before age twelve, experience somewhat elevated rates of breast cancer than do those who become sexually mature later. Women who reach menopause later than age fifty-five also have an increased risk of this disease. Presumably this is because these women are exposed for a longer period of time to whatever natural hormones may be involved in the causation of this disease. Women who have their ovaries removed before age forty have a significantly lower rate of breast cancer. Overall, surgical menopause is associated with a 40 percent reduction in risk.

While these three observations cannot help you right now in avoiding cancer, they do provide scientists with some useful clues. If the hormonal causation of breast cancer could be understood, women could be offered preventative measures. Already it is suggested that the synthetic hormones in the oral contraceptives may as an unexplained side effect be offering some slight protection against breast cancer.

MALE SEXUALLY RELATED CANCERS

Cancer of the penis is a very rare disease in the United States. It occurs most frequently in areas of the world where circumcision is not practiced and where penile hygiene is poor. Other than that, there is very little information about what causes this disease.

Prostate cancer, as we mentioned in the chapter on diet, is a leading cause of male cancer death in this country. Overrich diets, and the subsequent overstimulation of the gland by hormones, probably plays a more significant role than do sexual factors. But the few epidemiological studies that have been done in this area, do suggest that sexual activity might somehow be involved. Married men have higher rates of this disease than do unmarried men. One recent team of investigators reported that patients with prostatic cancer exhibited a greater sexual drive, suggesting that perhaps there is a venereally transmitted agent operative here. The fact that cervical cancer is reported more often among women married to men with prostatic cancer does suggest that there is a common cause.

Malignant tumors of the testes are not common. The cause is unknown, but it is generally accepted that trauma or sexual activity have nothing to do with these tumors. Some 15 percent of the cases occur in undescended testes—a rate forty-five times higher than in normal testes.

HOW TO PREVENT CANCER
(OR HELP YOUR CHILDREN TO DO SO)

For Females:

1. Postpone sexual intercourse until age eighteen or later. If intercourse does occur before that age, use a condom regularly.

2. If you have multiple sexual partners, always use a condom.

3. If it is practical, have your first child prior to age thirty.

4. Maintain high standards of personal hygiene—and make sure your sexual partner(s) does also.

For Males:

1. Consider circumcision at infancy to be a routine, desirable form of personal preventive health.

2. If you have multiple sexual partners, use a condom.

3. Maintain high standards of personal hygiene—and make sure your sexual partner(s) does also.

10

OCCUPATION

"The disease, in these people, seems to derive its origin from a lodgement of soot in the rugae of the scrotum. . . ."
            Percivall Pott, 1775,
            commenting on the unusual
            incidence of cancer of
            the scrotum among chimney sweeps

In this chapter and the one dealing with additives and pesticides, reference will be made to "parts per million." This is a very small amount of anything. To keep things in perspective remember that one part per million is equivalent to

—one inch in sixteen miles
—one minute in two years
—a one-gram needle in a ton of hay
—one penny in $10,000
—one ounce of salt in 62,500 pounds
—one large mouthful of food in comparison with the food a person will eat in a lifetime
—one drop of vermouth in 80 fifths of gin or vodka.

This unit of measure is often further subdivided to "parts per billion." One part per million is made up of 1,000 parts per billion.

During 1921, Phillip Hill, age twenty-three, began working at a dye manufacturing plant in New Jersey. In the course of his many tasks, he loaded vats with raw materials, operated machines and cleaned out the tanks once the processing was done. As a result he came in contact with a multitude of industrial chemicals.

Sometimes the fumes from the vats overwhelmed him. It was not unusual for his skin to come in contact with the various fluids he was mixing. Sometimes the solutions seeped through his shirt and pants.

During his twelve years at the plant, Phillip did not use any special type of protective clothing or equipment.

In 1933, he began to notice traces of blood in his urine. The blood appeared irregularly, present one day, gone the next. Soon thereafter, he suffered a noticeable weight loss, medium-grade fever and tenderness in the area of his bladder. Urination became frequent and it was increasingly accompanied by a painful burning sensation. A cystoscopic examination, where a small tube was inserted into his urethra revealed the presence of a large malignant tumor. Surgery was impractical. He died of industrially-induced bladder cancer at the age of thirty-six.

Stuart Murphy was one of a few hundred men and women who joined in the shipbuilding effort at the Long Beach Naval Shipyard in 1942.

He helped install asbestos insulation in the steam power plants. As he described it, "You would take the white stuff, make mud out of it, and throw it on the pipes."

Asbestos is an exceedingly dry material and working with it was often like being in the middle of a snowstorm. When conditions became particularly bad, Stuart would hold his breath as long as he could, but inevitably the asbestos cloud would outlast him and he ended up being forced to breathe deeply.

After working there for six months, Stuart quit, spent the next four years in the navy, returned to college and by 1950 was teaching high school physics in Chicago.

In 1966, twenty-four years after he spent six months at the shipyard, he experienced a persistent cough. He became breathless after walking up even one flight of stairs at school. Eventually, his breathing became so strained that he could be heard on the other side of the room.

An X ray showed heavy shadows in the lower two-thirds of his

lung field. Stuart's condition was diagnosed as diffuse pleural mesothelioma, a cancer induced by exposure to heavy amounts of asbestos. His physician informed him that because the condition
eventually covers the whole lung area, often infusing the entire ab-
domen, surgery was impossible. He could not remove all the dam-
aged organs and still have a surviving patient. Stuart was dead
within a year.

Marty Anderson joined the staff of a plastics manufacturing
group in the midwestern United States in 1959 when he was
twenty-two years old. He didn't have any particular education or
training, so he started at the bottom of the rung, accepting an as-
signment as a "pot cleaner."

The plastics materials were made from a colorless gas called
"vinyl chloride monomer" or VCM, for short, a substance derived
from chlorine and petroleum or natural gases. VCM is the raw material from which polyvinyl chloride (PVC) resin is made during a
process known as "polymerization." The resin is used to make plastic products. Once the vinyl chloride monomer was brought to the
plant, it was unloaded and piped in measured amounts into large
polymerization reactor vats. This was accomplished through an es-
sentially closed system. Marty and his associates did not have to
worry about coming in contact with VCM at that point. Then,
catalysts, emulsifiers and other chemicals were added to the VCM
gas in the vat, heat and pressure applied, and the reaction carried
out to its desired point. Then the polymerized material was
dropped into a secondary vat and the VCM gas which had not
reacted was recovered and recycled back through a closed system.
The polymerized material then entered a third set of tanks from
which it was dried and packaged. The end products in this third
tank were three different materials: first the PVC resin, a powder
of the texture of refined sugar; second a PVC paste, a very fine
powder with the texture of processed flour; and third, a PVC latex,
a stable suspension of PVC in liquid.

Up until this point in the polymerization process, Marty, or anyone else, did not come in contact with large amounts of vinyl chloride monomer or any other chemical.

But after the processing was complete, it was Marty's job (and
that of other pot cleaners) to open the reactor, climb into the six by

ten foot tank and with a hammer and chisel, chip the powder off the inside surface. Before he entered the tank, the air had been replaced a number of times, but nevertheless, when he opened the reactor it was not unusual for a burst of air, complete with particles of powder, to come in contact with his face momentarily. When he was in the tank doing his work, the only source of fresh air was a two-foot opening at the top. Sometimes as he chipped away at the powder, VCM gas which had been trapped within the powder during polymerization was released.

The job was dull, always messy, and sometimes it became very hot in the plant. Frequently Marty and his coworkers would take a break and cool off by throwing a cup or two of the vinyl chloride liquid on each other's back. It evaporated quickly—it was like pouring ether on your skin and the effect was refreshing.

Vinyl chloride is a colorless, faintly sweet-smelling gas at room temperature. Some of Marty's friends liked the smell and the anesthetic effect it had on them. They literally became hooked on the stuff and would sneak sniffs whenever they could.

Marty Anderson continued to work at the plant and in the mid-1960s was promoted to a more pleasant task.

He was in excellent health until 1973. Around that time, he noticed that his stools took on a tarlike shade of black. He consulted a physician who made a tentative diagnosis of "bleeding ulcer" and put him on a special diet.

But a few months later he returned, this time complaining of a vague pain in the upper right quadrant of his body. A physical exam showed that his liver was markedly enlarged, and a subsequent liver scan found a large lesion on the left lobe. Exploratory surgery confirmed that Marty had angiosarcoma, an extremely rare liver disease. He underwent cobalt treatment and after a stormy course recovered enough to return to work for a while. But in September of 1974, he succumbed to angiosarcoma. He was thirty-seven years old.

OCCUPATIONAL DISEASES

For centuries it's been known that certain occupations increase workers' risks of developing various diseases. Tragically, the association between the exposure and the risk was made after the fact, and human lives were lost.

The classic case of occupationally induced cancer is that reported by Percivall Pott in his book, *Chirurgical Observations,* which included a chapter entitled, "A Short Treatise of the Chimney Sweeper's Cancer." The chapter contained only 725 words, but the observations recorded in it provided the first clear description of an environmental cause of cancer, implied a way to prevent the disease, and led indirectly to the synthesis of the first known pure carcinogen. He described the plight of the chimney sweeps as follows:

> The fate of these people seems singularly hard; in their infancy, they are most frequently treated with great brutality, and almost, starved with cold and hunger; they are thrust up narrow, and sometimes hot chimnies, where they are bruised, burned, and almost suffocated; and when they get to puberty, become liable to a noisome, painful and fatal disease.

As Pott alluded, the sweeps were young boys who were kept on a minimal diet in an effort to keep them small, so they could physically enter the chimneys and do their most unpleasant task. Hygiene was very poor and in the course of their sweeping, soot accumulated on their scrotums. Pott had identified an environmental cause of scrotal cancer. In 1915 Japanese workers, Yamagiwa and Ichikawa supplied another part of the answer: they painted coal tar on a rabbit's ear and produced cancer. And in 1933 Cook and his associates put together the last piece of the puzzle: they identified the powerful carcinogen benzo(a)pyrene from coal tar.

In the 18th century, young boys cleaning chimneys were regularly exposing themselves to benzo(a)pyrene, and probably a series of other carcinogens.

The list of occupationally induced cancers is long and depressing. The increased incidence of "mountain disease," which turns out to be lung cancer, among those working in the uranium-rich mines of Schneeberg and Joachimsthal has already been mentioned. So has the case of the dial workers and early radiologists who succumbed to the hazards of their trade.

But there are many more examples: vineyard workers using arsenic sprays; smelters and others who came in frequent contact with high levels of inorganic arsenic manifest high rates of skin, lung, and liver cancers; shoemakers, who worked with a solvent containing a high percentage of benzene, had a very high rate of leukemia. Members of the chromate industry had an unusually high rate of cancer of the lung, nasal cavity, sinuses, and larynx. Workers coming in frequent contact with mustard gas had significantly higher mortality from cancer of the larynx, lung trachea, and bronchi than do most men. And the list goes on.

Occupationally induced diseases are sometimes rather difficult to identify. With ten or more years elapsing between exposure and the onset of the symptoms of the disease, the victim may be in a job totally unrelated to the one that caused his illness. He might not even remember that he was exposed to an industrial hazard. For instance, Stuart Murphy who worked for a brief time with asbestos in shipbuilding and then became a high school teacher would have no reason to suspect that that brief period of employment was the cause of his fatal disease. Making such a connection requires the skill of complete medical history taking and astute observation on the part of the diagnosing physician.

The three case histories—three of literally thousands of occupational cancer deaths which have occurred in the past three hundred years—are understandably frightening. One cannot help think, "Couldn't they have prevented them from happening?" "Couldn't they have known in advance that exposures to high levels of almost any industrial chemical might cause cancer?" And in terms of our own personal risks of developing cancer, you probably cannot help but wonder if the chemicals which proved lethal in the workplace could possibly escape and affect the general population.

A closer look at the facts behind the aromatic dyes, asbestos, and vinyl chloride stories might provide some partial answers to those questions.

AROMATIC DYES

Natural forms of coloring, for fabrics, cosmetics, food, have been used since ancient times. But because the supply of them was limited, the cost was extraordinarily high, and a spectrum of colors was out of reach of the average man.

In 1856, William Henry Perkin, while experimenting in his laboratory, discovered the pigments of what came to be known as the aniline group of dyes, and succeeded in producing a synthetic violet color. His discovery was received enthusiastically and by 1860, a thriving dye business was established in Germany.

Prior to World War I, Germany held a near monopoly on the "aniline dye" business. But just before and after the war, Switzerland, England, France—and the United States—established their own dye industries.

The first indication that exposure to the dyes in the course of the manufacturing process might have an adverse effect on human health came in 1895. In that year, Dr. Ludwig Rehn reported to the Congress of German Surgeons, that he had diagnosed three, possibly four cases of bladder tumors among forty-five men working in the manufacture of the chemical fuchsin. The dye-related compound fuchsin manufactured at the plant was prepared by mixing and heating a number of chemicals, including aniline and nitrobenzene. He felt that it was the inhalation of the aniline vapor that was causing the tumors.

Rehn's associates did not agree. They believed that he was making an unnecessary fuss. Those three tumors could have occurred by chance.

But by 1906, Rehn had diagnosed thirty-three additional cases from seven different factories and thus there was no more room for controversy. He wrote that in "the melting shop on hot days when there is much evaporation . . . of aniline and so on, new workmen are often so affected by urgency of micturition that urine passes involuntarily into their clothes."

In 1921, Phillip Hill began working at the dye manufacturing plant in the United States.

In the 1930s Dr. W. C. Hueper demonstrated that beta-2-naphthylamine, a dyestuffs intermediate, was a potent bladder carcinogen in the dog and one of at least four aromatic amines which were likely responsible for the causes of industrial bladder cancer which were now being diagnosed in dye workers with increased frequency. Dr. Ludwig Rehn was right about the risks associated with the manufacture of these dyes, although he was not at that time able to identify exactly what the carcinogenic chemical was.

Was It Preventable?

Given that the preliminary results as early as the late 1890s suggested that some aspect of the dye manufacturing process threatened human health—and this was repeatedly confirmed in the early part of the 1900s—it does seem odd that the first protective measures in the United States were not implemented until about 1930, *after* bladder tumors began to show up here.

It is always easy to be critical in retrospect, and we must acknowledge that the pace at which medical intelligence was circulated was nowhere near as fast as it is today—and the industrial technology available for reducing risk was not very sophisticated.

On the other hand, there is enough evidence to suggest that many of the small chemical companies around the United States—and those which used chemicals, for instance in the rubber industry—did do a great deal of foot-dragging in the area of keeping worker protection standards high. As late as 1955, some of the smaller outfits continued to maintain shockingly hazardous conditions, using highly dangerous chemicals in a promiscuous manner. Although federal guidelines had been set during the 1930s, there was not sufficient manpower to allow checking of every chemical manufacturer—and the smaller a company was, the less likely it was to be checked. Perhaps it is simply part of human nature not to conform to a new set of rules until you are prodded to do so.

For the most part, the large chemical plants, like E. I. du Pont, instituted and stuck with stringent worker protection protocols from 1930 on. But even they had problems keeping workers out of contact with carcinogens such as beta-naphthylamine, and because they felt that they could not deal with this chemical safely, they discontinued using it in 1956. Other suspected carcinogens were discontinued in the next few years. Most other large chemical companies followed suit, but again the smaller ones, although they knew the rules of the game, elected to play their way—at the cost of health and lives of some of their employees.

In 1978 occupational bladder cancers were still being diagnosed among employees of chemical companies around the country, cancers which are due to exposure to carcinogens during the mid-1950s. But the rate of new cases is now slacking off considerably, a reflection of the assumption—the hope—that the problem was solved by 1960.

Given that it was the intermediates of the aromatic dyes—that is, the chemicals that went into their preparations, not the dyes themselves—that caused cancer, there is no reason to believe that anyone outside the workplace was adversely affected by them through toxic fumes, contact with the clothes of a worker, or contact with the finished product.

ASBESTOS

Asbestos has been used for more than four thousand years. But up until one hundred years ago, when large-scale asbestos mining projects were first undertaken in Canada in a determined effort to counteract rising fuel costs by finding a new type of thermal insulation, it was considered more a treasure than a commercial raw material.

During the first century, deceased emperors were dressed in it prior to burial. Plutarch (A.D. 70) described how "asbesta" was used for wicks (the word *asbesta* means "unquenchable, inextinguishable or inconsumable"). Marco Polo in his famous diaries in the 13th century was fascinated with it, referring to asbestos as "a substance [which] when woven into cloth and thrown into the fire . . . remains incombustible."

The history of the adverse effect associated with the inhalation of asbestos also goes back to ancient times. The Roman naturalist Pliny the Elder mentioned in passing the sickness in the lungs of slaves whose occupation it was to weave asbestos into cloth. This was the first reference ever made to the disease now known as asbestosis.

The modern medical troubles of asbestos were recognized at the turn of the century, soon after the asbestos industry began to develop in North America and England. In 1900 Dr. H. Montague Murray at London's Charing Cross Hospital performed a post mortem examination on a thirty-three-year-old man who had worked for fourteen years in an asbestos textile factory. Dr. Murray found that the victim had been suffering from severe pulmonary fibrosis and noted specks of asbestos in the lung tissue.

In 1924, another English physician, Dr. W. E. Cook performed an autopsy on a thirty-three-year-old woman who had begun working at an asbestos textile plant at age thirteen. He also saw "curious bodies" in the lung, and designated it "asbestosis," a disease in which the asbestos particles interfere with the flow of oxygen to the blood.

Then, in 1935 Dr. Kenneth Lynch, a professor of pathology at the Medical College of South Carolina, reported a case of lung cancer in a fifty-seven-year-old asbestos worker. In 1946 a British team reported that 13 percent of the deaths among asbestos workers was due to cancer of the lung. Given that the impact of cigarette smoking was to be seen in later years, and lung cancer was a very rare disease, these results were highly significant.

In between these two dates, in 1942, Stuart Murphy worked for six months on asbestos insulation at the Long Beach Naval Shipyard.

During the 1950s and 1960s the evidence that incriminated asbestos inhalation with the very rare lung malignancy, mesothelioma, mounted steadily. In 1955, Dr. Richard S. Doll, Director of the Statistical Research Unit of the British Research Council, completed a study of 113 consecutive autopsies of men with more than twenty years exposure in a large asbestos-tile factory and found that they had a lung-cancer death rate eleven times as great as men in the general population of England and Wales.

During 1956 and 1957, Dr. J. Christopher Wagner at the Pneumoconiosis Research Unit of Johannesburg, South Africa, reported sixteen cases of a rare lung tumor known as mesothelioma, a disease which was not previously mentioned in medical books and not coded separately on the World Health Organization's International Classification of Diseases. These patients had been referred to this research center from a large asbestos mining area in the region. Could asbestos be involved?

Within a short period, cases of mesothelioma began to crop up elsewhere in South Africa and when Wagner and his associates discovered that the father of one of their new mesothelioma patients had been the manager of an asbestos mine and that the patient had played around in the mine and on the adjacent dumps as a child, they decided to obtain detailed life histories on all past and future victims of mesotheliomas. By the end of 1961, they had diagnosed a total of 89 cases of the malignancy. Only 12 of these proved to have had industrial exposure to asbestos, but all the rest came from the windswept region of the Cape's asbestos fields where they could easily have sustained exposure simply by living in the vicinity of asbestos mills and dumps.

In the mid-1960s Dr. Irving Selikoff, professor at the Mount Sinai School of Medicine and Director of its Environmental Laboratory, and Dr. E. Cuyler Hammond, Vice President for Epidemiology and Statistics at the American Cancer Society, did a follow-up study of men who worked in an asbestos-related job in 1942 (using records of union rosters of the International Association of Heat and Frost Insulators and Asbestos Workers). Taking the men's ages into account, Selikoff and Hammond calculated that 203 deaths could have been expected among the 632 men. Instead there were 255, an excess of 25 percent. The reason for the excess was not hard to find. Twelve deaths were attributed to asbestosis, 45 to cancer of the lung (where only 7 would be expected in a general male population this size). And where 9 or 10 gastrointestinal cancers were to be expected, there were actually 29.

Certainly cigarette smoking, which became increasingly popular in the 1940s and 1950s, played some role in that startling incidence of lung cancer. But even if all the asbestos workers were heavy smokers, that factor could not fully explain the observation. Later these same researchers showed that cigarette smoking enhanced the effects of asbestos (or vice versa) and that asbestos workers who smoked had a lung cancer rate 800 percent higher than did smokers in the general population.

Was It Preventable?

The evidence that asbestos inhalation posed a serious hazard to human health was accumulated very slowly during the first half of this century. It is easy to see how a nation at war, in desperate need of well-equipped ships, would put worker protection devices on a low priority, especially since they had no real reason to believe that working with asbestos posed a problem.

But with the accumulation of evidence throughout the 1950s and 1960s it is more difficult to understand why the problem was not taken more seriously. Many of the larger asbestos plants instituted protective measures in the 1950s. But some of the smaller ones were evidently very careless about human exposure to this known cancer-causing agent. A particularly infamous example was a plant in Tyler, Texas, which as late as 1970 was exposing its workers to asbestos levels sixty times or more higher than the currently accepted level.

As was the case with the aromatic dye industry, it seems that many of the earlier deaths were not preventable, in the sense that knowledge was so incomplete that a health risk was not recognized. But many asbestos plants were negligently slow in correcting matters—at the cost of the lives of many of their workers. The workers in some instances themselves often did not act to protect their own health, refusing to use the protective masks that were supplied.

Today industrial levels of asbestos are under strict government control, the limit in the plants being two fibers per cubic centimeter of air, where in early decades it often got as high as two hundred, three hundred, or more per cc. of air. Dust is sucked up through hoods over the machines and captured in a central bag house. The bagging is almost exclusively done now by machines. As an extra safety measure, many plants now hire only nonsmokers for certain jobs.

Asbestos and the General Public

One of the more frightening aspects of the asbestos story is the fact that the deaths recorded were not limited to one job category in one type of workplace. There were women who became victims of mesothelioma apparently simply because they regularly washed their asbestos-worker-husband's clothes; men and women who became victims because, as children, they played in a field contaminated with asbestos dust.

There is no doubt that asbestos is a frightening substance. Workers must be protected from its effects. We must do everything possible to eliminate its presence in our air. For instance, building demolition—which would tend to free asbestos fibers in their dry, deadly form, one in which they are easily inhaled—must be subject to strict controls.

VINYL CHLORIDE

Polymerization of the vinyl chloride monomer began in Germany in 1939. The United States became involved in its production some five years later. Polyvinyl chloride, much like asbestos, was hailed as a miracle substance—cheap, stable, fire-resistant, and able to assume an extraordinary range of soft and hard forms. Immediately it was designated for possible use in floor tiles, medical supplies, phonograph records, auto seat covers, wire insulations, and many other purposes.

Was it safe? During the 1940s, everyone seemed to think so. The primary worry then was the fire explosion potential of the gas. Once that was under control, the concerns were minimal.

In 1949, ten years after it was discovered, a Russian report indicated that a hepatitislike condition occurred in more than 25 percent of seventy-three polyvinyl chloride workers examined. The results of the report were circulated, but no one was terribly alarmed. During the 1950s, there were reports in many countries of a vaguely defined "vinyl chloride disease," the characteristics of which were nausea, dizziness, sometimes temporary loss of consciousness. Somewhat later were reports of a thickening of the skin at the finger tips, gradual dissolution of bone calcium at the fingertips, and heightened sensitivity to cold (collectively known as acroosteolysis), reported to occur in a small proportion of the workers involved in the manual cleaning of PVC reactors.

And also during the 1950s there were scattered industry-sponsored animal experiments which suggested that the vinyl chloride monomer in high doses might have some toxic effects—possibly affecting the liver. As a result, in the early 1960s the American Con-

ference of Governmental Industrial Hygienists, a voluntary stan-
dard-setting organization, put the maximum safe exposure level for
workers at 500 ppm.[1] Dow Chemical thought that was even too
high. When a 1961 animal experiment showed adverse liver effects
(but not cancer) in animals at doses as low as 100, they put an
upper limit at their plant at 50 ppm.

The reports of the local bone and skin reactions (acroosteolysis)
among a small number of pot cleaners led industry to do away with
the manual mechanism of pot cleaning. In the late 1960s they introduced high-pressure water hoses for cleaning, and only in rare
cases did men ever climb into the tanks again.

There was some concern about potential ill effects of some
aspects of the plastics production mechanism, so industry scientists made a voluntary commitment to keep testing vinyl chloride.

In May of 1970, at the 10th International Cancer Congress in
Houston, Texas, Dr. P. L. Viola of the Regina Elena Institute for
Cancer Research in Rome, Italy, and a medical director of Solvay
& Cie, a leading European PVC producer, reported that cancers
(but not angiosarcoma) in test animals could be produced at extremely high levels of exposure to vinyl chloride (10,000 to 30,000
ppm.). Dr. Viola concluded that there was "no implication to
human pathology" from this experiment, and no need to be concerned about workers exposed to less than 500 ppm. of the vinyl
chloride monomer. At that point, most PVC plants in the United
States were well below that level anyway.

In March of 1972, still eager to collect more data, seventeen
U.S. manufacturers of PVC and the VCM agreed to sponsor both
animal experiments and health studies in vinyl chloride monomer
workers in this country, the studies to be administered by the
Manufacturing Chemists Association. At the same time, the European industries were sponsoring similar animal tests, under the direction of Dr. Cesare Maltoni of the Instituto di Oncologia and
Centro Tumor in Bologna, Italy.

In January 1973, Dr. Maltoni came up with some disturbing
results. He detected a variety of tumors (including liver tumors) in
test animals subjected to concentrations of VCM as low as 250

1. Interestingly, this same level was accepted by the newly created Occupational
Safety and Health Administration (OSHA) in 1971.

ppm. In November 1973, Dr. Viola, who had previously been able to show malignant tumors at very high levels, confirmed that they could be induced at 250 ppm. The interest in the possible ill effects of vinyl chloride became more intense. But there was still no reason to believe that human health was threatened, even at high levels of exposure to the monomer.

Then in late 1973, Dr. John L. Creech, a local Louisville surgeon who helped oversee the health of B. F. Goodrich workers, casually mentioned to the Goodrich plant physician, Dr. Maurice N. Johnson, that he had recently seen two cases of a rare disease— angiosarcoma of the liver—one earlier that year and one about two years before. Dr. Johnson was startled, for he recognized this to be the same type of tumor that had been reported to occur in the Maltoni Rat Study. Angiosarcoma of the liver is a very rare disease, only some twenty-five to thirty cases being diagnosed each year in the U.S. When, a few weeks later, a third Louisville case of angiosarcoma came to their attention, they realized it was no coincidence. On January 22, 1974, the B. F. Goodrich Company notified employees, the National Institute of Occupational Safety and Health, and the Kentucky State Department of Labor that three of its workers had died from angiosarcoma of the liver.

This link was made by two astute physicians who, knowing that angiosarcoma was an extremely rare disease, concluded that there was some causal significance. Needless to say, if vinyl chloride caused a common tumor such as lung cancer, the picture would have been much less clear-cut and would have required many more cases and much more elaborate epidemiological manipulation to associate the tumor with the industrial exposure.

After the initial announcement, vinyl chloride plants outside Louisville began to examine their death records over the past ten years. Sometimes the cause of death was listed "primary liver cancer" or "liver cirrhosis," but eventually, it was established that the more likely cause was a liver angiosarcoma.

Within weeks of the discovery of the human cancer, Professor Maltoni of Italy found that tumors could be induced in animals at 50 ppm. But people hardly needed any more convincing then.

Even prior to the findings that the vinyl chloride monomer could cause cancer in workers exposed to high levels of it (note here that it is the *monomer*, or VCM, not the plastic resin, or PVC, which was linked with both human and animal tumors), federal regulatory agencies took action against the chemical. In 1973 and 1974 they banned various aerosol sprays which contained the monomer as a propellent. Similarly, once it was found that traces of the VCM could migrate from plastic liquor bottles to the alcohol, the government banned PVC plastic bottles for this use. (The primary concern here was that the taste of the liquor could be affected.) Ironically, not only were the VCM levels which migrated to the alcohol very small, but they would most likely have completely evaporated before the consumer had completed mixing his drink.

There was no reason to believe that either the aerosols or the use of VCM in the manufacture of liquor bottles ever posed a hazard whatsoever to human health, but in the interest of complete safety, the withdrawals were made. The industry did not oppose either move.

Could It Have Been Prevented?

With the state of technology that was available throughout the 1940s and 1950s, there was no way that scientists could have known that intense exposures to vinyl chloride monomer would cause human cancer. The moment that industry scientists became even slightly suspicious, protective measures were instituted and worker exposure levels were drastically lowered.

Although the animal experiments of the 1940s and 1950s were interesting, they were not alarming by any means. Many different chemicals, industrial or natural, will increase the incidence of tumors in test animals. When the early tests suggested that VCM in high doses affected animal tissues, the manufacturers did the only thing they could do—reduce worker exposure levels and keep testing.

Indeed it you compare the vinyl chloride story to that of asbestos and the aromatic dyes, you have a case of excellent industrial surveillance. Mount Sinai's Dr. Irving Selikoff calls the vinyl chloride incident a "success story": ". . . a success for science hav-

ing defined the problem, a success for labor in the rapid mobiliza-
tion of concern; success for government in urgently collecting data,
evaluating and translating it into necessary regulations; and success
for industry in preparing the necessary engineering control to minimize or eliminate the hazard."

Indeed it was the industry that supported all the studies. Ralph
L. Harding, Jr., president of the Society of the Plastics Industry,
Inc., summarized it: "This is a unique situation. Industry financed
the studies and industry blew the whistle on itself." But this fact is
often quickly forgotten by those who want to pin what was in most
respects an unavoidable tragedy on "evil industry."

PVC and VCM and the Public

The vinyl chloride episode was another frightening case of occupational disease, but again, it is easy to panic and lose perspective.

All authenticated cases of angiosarcoma occurred among workers engaged in closed environments during the conversion process
(polymerization) of the *vinyl chloride monomer* to polyvinyl chloride resin or in workers directly handling the monomer. A variety
of estimates put the *minimal* amount of exposure leading to disease
at between 200 and 500 ppm.—probably more. The average
length of worker exposure was seventeen years; the shortest period of exposure, four years.

Although press reports indicate otherwise, a government survey
of angiosarcoma deaths in the U.S. between 1964 and 1974 concluded that there was "no evidence that living around a vinyl chloride plant is a risk factor in the occurrence of liver angiosarcoma."[2]

Simply because intense levels of exposure to the vinyl chloride
monomer increased risks of this rare form of liver cancer among
plant workers, does *not* mean that the polyvinyl chloride resin is
cancer-causing. Even more important, the plastic products themselves—for instance, automobile seats and phonograph records,

2. Recent press reports also indicated that wives of PVC and VCM workers were
more likely than other women to have children with birth defects, and to suffer miscarriages. As of this writing, there is no evidence to back up either of these claims.

which are many stages removed from the monomer and the polyvinyl chloride resin—pose no health threat. The "new-car smell," for instance, has nothing to do with VCM or PVC.

Application of heat to plastic products does *not* lead to the depolymerization of the PVC back to the chloride gas.

Prior to the disclosure that a small number of workers exposed to VCM had developed a rare form of liver cancer, the plastics industry did a significant amount of research to ensure that even small amounts of the vinyl chloride monomer were not present in wraps that came in contact with food. During the 1960s and for the first couple of years of the 1970s, there were trace amounts of the monomer in some food wraps, certainly not enough to cause any harm, but the fact that any detectable amounts were there raised eyebrows at the Food and Drug Administration. Our current laws state that intentionally added food additives *and* nonintentional food additives which may migrate to food from wrappings cannot contain a substance which has been shown in any amounts to induce cancer in any laboratory animals.

As of now, there is no reasonable risk posed to the individual who uses plastic wrap or plastic containers. At the very most, if one had highly sensitive techniques (which we do not have), you might find trace amounts at the level of a few parts per *billion* of vinyl chloride monomer in some of the rigid or semirigid plastic food materials. But then, if you tested long and hard enough, you could probably find anything in anything. This level is not of practical significance.

But, nevertheless, in July of 1975, the Ralph Nader associated Health Research Group petitioned the FDA to ban completely all polyvinyl chloride food packaging materials. The FDA responded shortly thereafter indicating that they would permit continued use of the plasticized "film" for wrapping meats and other food products, but would reevaluate the use of rigid polyvinyl chloride bottles and thick wrap such as blister packs. This distinction was based on the fact that while thin wrap is completely processed and the monomer completely removed, the rigid and semirigid type might have traces of the monomer. But again, for all practical purposes the monomer is *not* present in these containers.

As of this writing, the "reevaluation" is still in process and it remains possible that in the atmosphere of panic surrounding the PVC and VCM issues, the FDA may overreact, feeling that they should "do something" and ban rigid plastics even without cause. Recently the Council on Wage and Price Stability, seeing the economic implications of this move and the inevitable rise in consumer prices, urged them not to do so, writing that such action may be "unnecessary or may be more restrictive than is required to prevent the ingestion of vinyl chloride."

You may think, "Oh, we can live without plastic bottles for our salad dressing and vegetable oil and there must be something else to cover luncheon meats." But the fact is that plastic food wraps have revolutionized the food distribution system in this country, and this is reflected in both lower costs and tremendous variety in our supermarkets.

OCCUPATIONAL CANCER: A PERSPECTIVE:

We've learned a great deal about occupational causes of cancer in the past three decades. But the subject is still relatively new, and we are still groping with means of how to handle them. On one hand, some people maintain that human life is more important than any industry or any product, and that if a problem comes up, the item or items involved should be banned. On the other hand, other individuals, while agreeing that the protection of human life is the number one priority, point out there are safe ways of using unsafe materials and that we could institute effective protective measures for exposed workers, and base our actions and consider the issue in terms of six general guidelines.

First, while it is acknowledged that under some circumstances, high levels of occupational chemicals can cause human cancer, this does not automatically mean that low amounts of them—even traces—also pose a cancer risk. Certainly the fact that a human carcinogen shows up in some aspect of our environment should stimulate action. For instance, when asbestos traces were found in the water supply of Duluth, Minnesota, and New Orleans, Louisiana, that was a source of legitimate concern, even though we have no reason to believe that small amounts of ingested asbestos would have anything like the effects of high levels of inhaled asbestos. Nevertheless, it is something that should be investigated, and steps taken to reduce as much as possible the level of the chemical. It should not, however, incite panic. The disease statistics in both those cities offer no basis for suspecting that asbestos in water is causing disease or death.

Second, it is critical that in discussing occupational disease, we not exaggerate the situation. In total, less than thirty United States workers have thus far died from VCM-induced angiosarcoma of the liver. But given the headline space the topic has been given, many people think the number is more like thirty thousand. Perhaps some 200 or 250 Americans have died as a result of exposure to asbestos, and, over the years, some 500 or 600 due to industrial carcinogens that caused bladder cancer. This is not to minimize the tragedy of the men and women who were involved. It is to lend some perspective to the extent of the problem we are dealing with.

Third, the chemicals we have discussed in this chapter pose, except in some very rare circumstances, a negligible risk to you unless you are working in an industrial situation which puts you in frequent contact with chemicals, and pose only a relatively small risk to the industrial workers themselves. Dr. John Higginson, Director of the International Agency for Research on Cancer, has estimated that a nonsmoking asbestos worker exposed to certain types of asbestos may possibly increase his risk of death by age sixty-five from 30 to 33 per 100, or by between 2 and 3 percent, due to mesothelioma. The risks of dying from angiosarcoma following high exposure to vinyl chloride monomer are dubious due to the scanty data available. But Dr. Higginson, assuming that there is a four-hundred-fold greater risk of exposed workers, has calculated that an individual increases his chance of dying before age sixty-five by between 0.3 and 0.4 percent, the equivalent to smoking three cigarettes a day for fifteen years. The risk is very small in comparison to that of lung cancer in a heavy smoker, where the risk is at least twenty times greater.

Fourth, most diseases identified with industrial causes are also caused by other factors.

For instance, lung cancer risk is increased with exposure to asbestos. But many people associated with the asbestos business or living in an area near an asbestos plant die from lung cancer because they smoke cigarettes, not because of exposure to the fiber. Some workers in the chemical industry and those living in the immediate vicinity develop bladder tumors spontaneously, and as a result of cigarette smoking, not because of occupational carcinogens. Angiosarcoma is such a rare disease, that the analogy is not as appropriate here, but even in this case, rare liver disturbances do occur outside an occupational setting. In the months following the disclosure of the Goodrich VCM worker deaths, there were scattered reports of angiosarcoma of the liver deaths in areas near the plant. Subsequent investigations indicated that these had nothing to do with polymerization of plastic materials, but were rather the results of better diagnosis, that is, with angiosarcoma in the newspapers constantly, physicians became more familiar with its symptoms and where, under other circumstances, they might have listed a cause of death as "liver cancer," they were then more specific.

Fifth, although tragedies have been associated with certain occupational chemicals, we can't forget that many of these very same chemicals have saved more lives than they took. For instance, in the furor over asbestos, many people forget that the "miracle fiber" was used to prevent fires, to make auto brakes safer. In discussing the much-maligned plastics, one can overlook its indispensable use in the medical field—blood bags and medical tubing which has saved thousands of lives. On another level, we have to remember that banning plastic bottles because of some hypothetical cancer risk will inevitably lead to more home accidents, some quite serious, from broken glass.

Sixth, we are not dealing here with an "us versus them" situation. When it comes to industrial production in the United States, we are all in this together. We all benefit from the lifesaving and simply pleasurable aspects of modern living. While federal regulation and surveillance of employee working conditions in chemical plants—and in work environments which use chemicals—is obviously necessary, it is pointless to accuse an industry of deliberately using human life to their own advantage in making profits.

That is an accusation more appropriate to the early part of this century, not the 1970s. On the other hand, it is clear that there is an ongoing need for monitoring the various chemical industries to ensure that established regulations are followed and that workers' health is not impaired by exposure to toxic or carcinogenic chemicals.

HOW TO PREVENT CANCER:

1. If you work in a chemical plant, or in an environment in which you are exposed to industrial chemicals, *always* follow the safety instructions of your plant. At least some of the occupational tragedies of the past were due to workers being careless about their own health.

2. Be extremely cautious in tearing down parts of a house, shed, or other structure that could be lined with asbestos. Be particularly careful when you encounter insulation material which may well contain significant amounts of dry asbestos.

PART II

Some Much-Talked-About Factors Which Have Never Been Shown to Increase Your Odds on Developing Cancer

11

"CHEMICALS" IN FOOD

"Sola dosis facit venenum" [Only the dose makes the poison].
                    Paracelus, a Renaissance physician.

If you asked the average American today to list three things that "caused cancer" the odds are that he or she would include both food additives and pesticide sprays.

The bannings or proposed bannings of food-coloring agents, artificial sweeteners, cattle-growth stimulants, meat and fish curing products, and pesticides have caused a great deal of anxiety about these chemicals. Tragically, the panic over additives and pesticides has almost completely obscured dissemination about a more likely food-related cancer risk, namely the ingestion of overly rich diets.

The chemicals discussed in this chapter are classified as "hypothetical risks" because, in contrast to the eight known risks described in the first part of this book, there is no evidence that in the manner they are used, they caused or played any role in the 385,000 cancer deaths which occurred in the United States last year.

FOOD ADDITIVES AND PESTICIDES

Our knowledge about the causes of human cancer rests almost exclusively on studies of differences in disease patterns between various human populations.

For example, the fact that the breast and colon cancer-rates are relatively high in this country and relatively low in Japan led us to attempt to identify the factor which distinguishes these two countries might explain the difference in cancer incidence. Differential intake of dietary fats emerged as the most likely explanation.

So in considering food additives and pesticides, we might also start with some epidemiological considerations. If man-made food chemicals did play some role in cancer causation, then non-Western countries where modern agricultural and food processing techniques are not widespread might be expected to have lower rates of cancer. Similarly, given that food additive use has increased in this country in the last sixty years and, allowing for a twenty-year latency period for cancer development, you might expect to see an increase in one or more forms of cancer death in the past forty years. If there were an increase and we were to make a case for the role of food additives and pesticides, that increase in disease would have to occur in both sexes.

The arguments in favor of food additives as carcinogens fail on both points. First, countries like Poland and Czechoslovakia, which do not use our means of food production or preservation, have overall cancer death rates which are similar to or higher than ours. Second, U.S. trends in cancer mortality offer no evidence that additives or pesticides increased the number of cancer deaths in the past four decades.

The male death rate from lung cancer has increased by more than twenty-five times since 1930. Even the most avid natural foods advocate would not maintain that additives or pesticides cause lung cancer. There has been no great difference in mortality from cancer of the breast, colon-rectum, esophagus, oral cavity, thyroid, or uterus in the past forty years. There has been an increase in the incidence of bladder cancer in men, but not in women and given that there is no difference to exposure to food and agricultural chemicals by sex, that rules out a role for them there.

If food chemicals were involved, you might think they would have the stomach as at least one of their targets. In the years following the stepped-up use of food additives and pesticides, there has been a *steady decrease* in the incidence and death rate from stomach cancer in both sexes.

But the focus on additives and pesticides as possible carcinogens has not been on human cancer statistics, but on animal experiments. The food safety laws in the United States, specifically, the so-called Delaney Clause, part of the 1958 Food Additives Amendment, are such that a food additive or pesticide can be banned if just one animal experiment reports that some type of cancer has been associated with its use. The Delaney Clause states that:

> No additive shall be deemed to be safe if it is found to induce cancer when ingested by man or animal, or if it is found, after tests which are appropriate for the evaluation of the safety of food additives, to induce cancer in man or animals. . . .[1]

In other words an additive or pesticide can make headlines as a "cancer-causing agent" if one group of mice fed large doses of it develops tumors. This does *not* mean that the chemical in question causes or has ever caused any form of human cancer. When the cancer-causing effect is limited to just one species of animal—as is generally the case in the examples below—it does not even suggest that it *might* cause human cancer. What would be alarming would be the observation that a chemical led to an increased incidence of tumors in, for instance, the mouse, rat and dog. But the way the laws are written, evidence gathered from one species—indeed, even one cancer-prone strain of mice—is sufficient grounds for banning a chemical. (Some of the specific problems of the Delaney Clause will be discussed in Chapter 14).

But the issue here is less the appropriateness of our food laws, and more an interest in the possible role additives and pesticides play in cancer. It has already been established that there is no evidence from studies of human populations that these factors are

1. Food Additives Amendment of 1958, Section 409(c)(3)(A) 21 U.S.C. Section 348(c)A 1964.

playing a role in U.S. cancer deaths. The next step is to see what types of animal evidence are available.

By the time a chemical gets through all the types of preclearance testing it must before being allowed in our food supply, it is, by our current standards, safe. There are chemicals which are considered for use in these roles and rejected because of preliminary evidence that they could pose a threat. But you never hear of them. They never get to a research stage which would merit their attention. Ironically, the ones you do hear the most about, are the ones that have been most thoroughly studied. Below are a few examples of the facts behind the myths that pesticides, additives and other environmental chemicals "cause cancer."

PESTICIDES

In November 1959, large quantities of cranberries were destroyed because they had been sprayed with the "cancer-causing agent" aminotriazole. On Thanksgiving day that year, many people were concerned enough about all cranberry sauce that they omitted the item from their menu (but, of course, many lit up cigarettes after their cranberry-less dinner).

Since 1959 many other pesticides have been indicted as human cancer risks but in general, the evidence is as flimsy as the evidence against food additives.

DDT, aldrin, and dieldrin have all been banned. In the case of DDT, the banning allegedly was based on the report that it caused wild birds to lay eggs with soft shells, thus interfering with reproduction, an allegation which is still, in the opinion of many scientists, unsubstantiated. DDT, aldrin, and dieldrin all cause liver tumors in mice and it was this factor that led to the demise of these two pesticides, and was a major part of the "rationale" calling for a ban on DDT.

In making the decision that aldrin and dieldrin were "imminent hazards," the Environmental Protection Agency overlooked the facts that phenobarbitol, a widely used drug which is taken in significantly higher dose levels than the traces of pesticides that may

show up on food, also causes liver tumors; that the mouse is generally considered to be an inappropriate test model for the purpose
of predicting carcinogenic response in man;[2] that aldrin and dieldrin did not cause cancer in other animals, for instance the dog;
and that men who had worked closely with these chemicals for
many years, being exposed to levels many hundred times that of
the general population, did not have unusually high rates of any
form of cancer.

In the last five years, many people have assumed a "since they
might cause cancer, we can live without them" attitude toward
pesticides. We are such an agriculturally advanced country that it
is easy for a moment to forget that man has traditionally struggled
to protect himself from the ravages of pests, and that in many parts
of the world pesticides perform a lifesaving function. Speaking specifically, Dr. Philippe Shubik of the Eppley Institute for Research
in Cancer at the Nebraska Medical Center calls DDT "one of the
most useful compounds ever invented by mankind, perhaps second, or even parallel to, the antibiotics in lifesaving. Through
mosquito control alone, DDT is credited with having saved 10
million lives, prevented 200 million illnesses from malaria, yellow
fever and other diseases."

In our country where malaria is not a problem, we are depen-
dent on pesticides for agricultural efficiency—which translates to
low-priced food. We can do without a few pesticides but we can't
do without all of them. Continued banning of agricultural chemicals on the basis of evidence of cancer in one type of animal cannot
continue if we are to maintain our current large and varied food
supply.

Pesticides are by their very nature highly toxic in concentrated
form. If misused they can cause ill health in man. The recent incident involving the pesticide kepone, which left thirty people
hospitalized with tremors, blurred vision, loss of memory, steril-
ity, and the possibility of liver damage, exemplifies what can hap-

2. The World Health Organization Expert Committee on Pesticide Residues reported, in regard to use of mice in making judgments, that "it would be unwise to
classify a substance as a carcinogen solely on the basis of evidence of an increased incidence of tumors of a kind that may occur spontaneously with such a high
frequency."

pen when individuals are careless in the use of such powerful chemicals.

We need to regulate and oversee pesticide use. But there is no reason to suspect that any pesticide in past or present use has caused or will cause human cancer. The level of pesticide residues is carefully monitored and are generally found to be significantly lower than that allowed by law. Two major scientific groups have recently evaluated the pesticide issue and reached similar conclusions: The National Academy of Science has stated that "the evidence is that the United States does have a good set of laws governing the manufacture, sale and use of pesticides and that they are being administered to give protection to both the public and the environment." In 1973 the President's Panel on Chemicals and Health flatly stated that "there is no evidence from human experience that pesticides currently in use have been the cause of cancer . . . in man."

"Tris" and "Cancer Causing Chemicals" in Plastic Bottles

In 1973, the federal government banned the sale of flammable children's nightwear because of the concern about fire deaths. The garment industry under pressure from regulatory groups to use flame retardants at that point began to use increasing amounts of "tris" (2,3,dibromopropyl) phosphate. As of 1977 it was estimated that some 35 to 40 percent of children's sleepwear had been treated with this substance.

Recently, following the report that tris could induce cancer in rats and mice, it was claimed in various press reports that this chemical could be responsible for thousands of cases of childhood cancers, particularly kidney cancer.

Whether or not tris should be banned is a question to be settled after laboratory evidence is reevaluated *and* after alternative means of ensuring that clothing can be made safely fireproof are identified. But what is clear is that the tris example is just another in a line of panic reactions following the announcement of results from animal experiments. There is no evidence from human studies that tris has caused any harm to health, although in the emotional atmosphere surrounding the discussion of this issue, that point seems to be lost.

Around the same time, another health scare emerged, this one relating to the use of plastic bottles to carry soft drinks like Coke. The particular concern was over acrylontrile, the fear being that this substance which can in high doses induce cancer in laboratory animals, could leak from the structure of the bottle. (This leaking occurs in rather unique circumstances, when the bottle is exposed to desert temperatures of 120-degrees Fahrenheit for six months). Again, whether or not acrylontrile should be used in bottling soft drinks is not the issue here (the manufacturers argue that the migration of the substance into the drink is at such a low level that it is not a "food additive" within the terms of the law), but what is, is the fact that Americans were worrying over yet another hypothetical risk instead of focusing on real ones which do indeed threaten their health.

NITRATES, NITRITES

The use of nitrates and nitrites in preparing bacon and in curing various meats recently has raised more anxieties than any other food additives.

The source of concern is that nitrates are capable of converting to nitrites, and nitrites can, when they combine with substances known as amines, produce nitrosamines. Nitrosamines have been shown to be strong carcinogens in most animals. Traces of nitrosamines have been found in some processed meats and a number of studies of cooked bacon found between 30 and 106 ppm. nitrosamines.

If you are concerned about bacon and other cured products posing a cancer risk, consider the following factors.

First, natural nitrates are found (often in levels exceeding 3,000 ppm.) in many vegetables, including spinach, beets, radishes, eggplant, celery, lettuce, collards, and turnip greens. These natural nitrates have the potential, under some circumstances, to convert externally or internally to nitrite. This natural nitrite is chemically identical to the nitrite used in curing meats.

Second, nitrite is a component of human saliva. A person gener-
ates approximately as much nitrite in his own saliva in a day as he
would consume from three meals in which cured meats were the
main course. Dr. Jonathan White from the United States Department of Agriculture estimates that about two-thirds of the average
American's intake comes from his own saliva, the other third from
cured meats.

Third, nitrates and nitrites are added to products for a purpose:
they prevent the development of deadly botulism-causing agents.
At this time, there is no other known way to assure the safety of
cured products. They are not "merely cosmetic," although they do
also impart a reddish color. Additionally, nitrite is essential for the
production of bacon, ham, frankfurters, and other cured meats. If
nitrites were not used, bacon would become salt pork, ham would
become salty roast pork, and frankfurters would be bratwurst.

The fact that nitrosamines are powerful carcinogens in animals,
and the suggestion that in some parts of the world alcoholic beverages which are contaminated with substantial amounts of naturally
occurring nitrosamines might contribute to cancer of the esophagus[3] are alarming and we should do everything possible to
keep nitrosamines out of our food supply. For example, nitrite
levels in bacon should be kept as low as possible. Evidence is now
accumulating that the use of ascorbic acid (vitamin C) in the curing
process may suppress the development of potentially dangerous
nitrosamines (having a glass of orange juice with your bacon might
have the same effect). But right now we are left with the following
conclusions: there is no reason to believe that nitrite-treated foods
cause cancer in the United States; there *is* reason to be concerned
enough about the nitrite-nitrosamine matter to warrant intensive
new research—any chemical which causes cancer in as many animal species as do nitrosamines is worthy of our immediate attention; but any restrictive or corrective actions, if they are instituted
at all, should encompass *all* exposure to nitrites—that in saliva
and vegetables, not just those in cured meats.

3. There is no confirmed evidence that links nitrites or nitrosamines with cancer
in man. But on the other hand, no animal species is fully resistant to carcinogenesis
by these compounds and therefore there is no reason to believe that man should not
be susceptible if nitrosamines were ingested at high enough dose levels for long
periods of time.

Red Dye #2

Red #2, or amaranth, was the most widely used food coloring in this country (it was found in soft drinks, ice cream, candy, baked goods, and elsewhere) until it was banned in early 1976.

The way it was reported in the press, it would appear that this coloring was being used for years without any knowledge of its health effect on animals. Indeed, just the opposite was true. A whole series of tests including five chronic feeding studies, two in rats, two in mice, and a seven-year study in dogs, were part of the original petition for the use of this color additive. Since 1970, at least nineteen scientific studies related to the safety of Red #2 have been carried out. Prior to the banning, only two Russian studies indicated that the coloring in high doses could bring about cancer. The other seventeen studies—which were performed on a number of different animals, including rats, mice, rabbits and hamsters—did *not* show cancer.

A great deal of publicity was given to the "mixed up" FDA study, and in the course of the subsequent scramble to get "more information" about the coloring, twenty years of evidence was put aside.

Red #2 was finally banned when a federally sponsored study suggested there was an increased incidence of tumors in rats which were fed so much of the dye it was surprising that they all didn't turn red. But again, there was never any evidence that the dye caused either human cancer or malignances in more than one type of animal.

DES

DES, the abbreviation for diethylstilbestrol, is a synthetic estrogen which has been used since 1954 as a cattle-growth stimulant. DES, the same chemical discussed in Chapter 9, which was used extensively during the 1940s in an attempt to prevent miscarriage, and led to the development of a rare form of vaginal cancer in a small number of the daughters of the women treated.

Its impact on cattle growth is very significant: a 500-pound animal being treated with DES will reach a marketable weight of 1,000 pounds in thirty-four days less time, using 500 pounds less feed than would an animal not receiving DES. Additionally, DES causes an increase of 7 percent in protein and moisture in meat, while resulting in a decrease in fat. The FDA estimates that the banning of DES would cost consumers about $500 million annually but others estimate a range from $800 million to one billion dollars.

The question here is, does DES, which has been shown to cause cancer when used as a drug during pregnancy, pose a threat to human health when it is used to stimulate cattle growth? A number of points are relevant.

First, DES is an estrogen, and both natural and artificial forms of estrogen have been shown to increase cancer risk in animals. But it is not the only source of estrogen to which American eaters are exposed. Milk, eggs, and honey have estrogen. It has been estimated that there is one thousand times the amount of estrogen in an egg than there is in a serving of beef liver from an animal treated with DES. Additionally, the oral contraceptive has far more synthetic estrogen than would a serving of liver with DES traces. Dr. Thomas Jukes of the University of California at Berkeley has noted that in a meal of ground round steak from DES-implanted cattle, whole wheat bread, mashed potatoes, green peas, and salad, the food containing the smallest amount of estrogen would be the meat. (Synthetic estrogens have no known biological activity lacking in natural estrogens.)

Second, a woman's body regularly produces estrogen. *Nature* estimated that it would take five hundred pounds of liver containing 2 parts per billion of DES to be equivalent (in terms of DES quantity) to the daily production of estrogen by a reproductive-age woman.

Third, although you hear about "DES, a cancer-causing agent in meat," the fact is that the traces of the hormone have only been found in the *liver* of the animal, not in the rest of the meat.

Fourth, the traces we're talking about are often in the fractions of a part per billion. Only the most highly sensitive tests could detect them. Women who were formerly treated with estrogen to prevent miscarriage received 5 to 125 milligrams for thirty or more consecutive weeks. To ingest a dose of just 50 mg. of DES, you would have to, at one sitting, eat twenty-five tons of beef liver containing 2 parts per billion DES.

Fifth, an arbitrary banning of DES would overlook its benefits. The most obvious is the economic savings—in terms of grain supply and beef availability at a lower cost. Less obvious, however, at least to the general population, is that the use of DES increases carcass protein and moisture and decreases carcass fat. *Given the growing evidence that fat in the diet increases the risk of various forms of cancer, the use of DES, instead of being a cancer risk, might indeed have an anticarcinogenic impact on our population.*

The issue of using or banning DES in cattle production has become a very emotional one. For our purposes, though, there is no reason whatsoever to think that eating meat from animals treated with DES poses a cancer threat. Again, we should be more concerned about eating large amounts of high-fat-content meats and liver (the latter because of its extraordinarily high cholesterol content), in particular, than about the cattle-growth stimulant.

ARTIFICIAL SWEETENERS

Cyclamates

Sodium and calcium cyclamates are salts of cyclamic acid (cyclohexysulphamic acid). For those with chemical phobia, the name might be enough to deter them. But then again, if you knew that a natural product like an egg contained zeaxanthine, butyric and acetic acids and conalbumin, you might feel the same way.

Cyclamates were discovered by Dr. Michael Sveda in 1937 while he was working in a laboratory at the University of Illinois. Before the sweetener was introduced by Abbott Laboratories in 1951, it passed a series of systematic safety tests, and when the list of "generally recognized as safe" (the so-called GRAS list) was drawn up in 1958, cyclamates were included.

Cyclamates first encountered trouble in June of 1959 when a University of Wisconsin study found that tumors developed in some white Swiss mice when cyclamate and cholesterol pellets were implanted in their bladders. But that test was considered inappropriate because the animals did not eat the sweetener. Then in the fall of that year, after eighteen years of intensive research which revealed no cancerous growths, the results of an industry-sponsored feeding study became available: of 240 rats eating a cyclamate-saccharin mixture, 8 of those at the highest dose levels developed what appeared to be bladder tumors. All the inevitable "experts" were called in—and all had their own different opinion about what they saw. As a *Lancet* editorial described it, "Never have so many pathologists been summoned to opine on so few lesions from so humble a species as the laboratory rat." But eventually all did agree that at least four of the tumors were carcinomas.

On October 18, 1969, then HEW Secretary, Robert H. Finch, announced that the findings of this single study required him to act in accordance with the Delaney Clause and terminate the usage of cyclamates in food products.

In the years following the banning of cyclamates, a battery of new tests were done and cyclamates, as they had prior to the fall of 1969, came out "clean." There is probably not one scientist in the United States who is familiar with the facts who now thinks that the sweetener should have been banned. Although it may take a court battle, the cyclamates may be back on our tables, and in our soft drinks, within the next four years.

Saccharin

Saccharin (from the Latin word for sugar, *saccharum*) is a white crystalline powder with a chemical appellation which also would make anyone with even a touch of chemical phobia shiver: 2,3,di-hydro-3-oxobenzisosulfonazole.

Its sweetening capacity was discovered—quite accidently—by Dr. Constantin Fahlberg, a German organic chemist, while working in his Johns Hopkins laboratory during the summer of 1879. He spattered a bit of an unknown compound on his hand, diluted it, and then, contrary to the basic rules of good laboratory practice, licked his fingers. The compound tasted sweet. Indeed, as was later shown, saccharin offers a sweetening power three hundred to five hundred times that of cane sugar. (Ironically, in its highly concentrated form this very sweet substance is exceedingly bitter.)

The commercial interest in the Fahlberg discovery was almost immediate. Saccharin was tried as an antiseptic, then as a preservative to inhibit fermentation in food. And during the 1880s it was introduced as a sugar substitute for diabetics. In 1907, food processors began to express an interest in adding it to fruits and vegetables. Thus sweet corn could be even sweeter without the caloric effects of sugar.

The question of saccharin's safety was raised soon after its discovery. After all,, it was a new "laboratory concoction" and certainly could not be assumed to be as innocuous as some naturally occurring substance. So, it was tested. Back in the 1880s and early 1900s, however, the subjects of safety experiments were not animals but humans. The first reports from Europe indicated the volunteers who ate large doses of the sweetener showed no untoward effects. (The interest at this point, of course, was in short-term effects, as opposed to the possible long-term, chronic effects which concern us today.)

But when saccharin was proposed as an additive for food in this country, the investigation became more intense. Then Chief Chemist, Dr. Harvey Wiley, established what came to be known as "the poison squad," a group of healthy young men to whom he fed heaping spoonfuls of various food additives. If these healthy human specimens survived the overdoses, Wiley reasoned, any moderate consumer certainly could not suffer ill effects. By 1907 Dr. Wiley was condemning saccharin in the presence of President Theodore Roosevelt because he had established, with the help of the poison squad, that very high doses of the artificial sweetener could cause loss of appetite, nausea, pressure in the stomach, and a general disturbance of "digestive functions." It was for these reasons that Wiley mounted a campaign to keep saccharin out of foods. But, interestingly, he approved its used for one purpose—sweetening chewing tobacco.

Owing in part to the efforts of President Roosevelt, Dr. Wiley was soon overruled and saccharin was approved for use in food and drugs (for example, in toothpastes). But in comparison to today's consumption patterns, the use was very limited. The shortages of sugar during the two World Wars brought temporary surges in saccharin consumption, but actually it was not until the late 1950s and early 1960s that artificially sweetened foods and drugs became really popular among the general public.

In the early 1950s the first toxicological studies on the safety of saccharin, using rats and mice, were conducted (by today's standards, these tests were neither sophisticated nor intensive). A review of these safety studies was made in 1955 by a committee appointed by the National Academy of Sciences. Their conclusion was that the sweetener in moderate doses posed no hazard either to animal or human health. There were two or three isolated laboratory experiments during the 1950s which found that exceedingly high doses of saccharin, either fed in the diet or implanted through pellets in the bladder, could increase the incidence of what appeared to be bladder tumors, but this was not considered a source of concern, the common interpretation being that the mere irritation caused by such large quantities of a chemical could account for the appearance of tumors.

Thus, since there was no known reason for concern about the safety of saccharin (or for that matter, about the safety of the sweetener cyclamates, introduced in 1951), artifically sweetened foods and beverages became more and more popular, despite the fact that the products were first introduced for those people who, for medical reasons, had to limit their sugar intake. Mothers saw saccharin-sweetened products as an effective way for reducing their children's sugar intake and, they hoped, the dentist's bills. Diet-conscious Americans saw saccharin products as a means of satisfying their cravings for sweets while keeping their waistlines.

The widespread use of both saccharin and cyclamates caused the National Academy of Sciences and other scientific research groups to look more closely at the sweeteners. Were they safe? Repeated animal studies could detect no problems. In 1967 the Food Protection Committee of the National Academy of Sciences reported to the Food and Drug Administration that one gram or less of saccharin per day (approximately the equivalent of seven 12-ounce bottles of diet soda or 60 small saccharin tablets) posed no hazard to adult health. But in the interest of assuring even greater confidence in saccharin safety, the Committee recommended further animal studies to determine if there was any previously undetected cancer-causing impact of the chemical on the internal organs of laboratory animals.

Then, in the fall of 1969 there was a dramatic change in the artificial sweetener picture in this country. As a result of the previously mentioned experiment which found that 8 of 240 rats eating a cyclamate-saccharin mixture developed what seemed to be bladder tumors, cyclamates were precipitously banned. As already noted, the underlying reason for this banning was the existent of the now-famous Delaney Clause, which requires that an additive shown to cause cancer in any animal experiment in any dose must be removed from the market.

Strangely, saccharin managed to maintain its status on the list of Generally Recognized as Safe food additives (the GRAS list), despite its complicity in the experiment indicting cyclamates as a cancer-causing agent. The Food and Drug Administration (FDA), or anyone else, has never adequately explained how an experiment involving more than one chemical (indeed, three chemicals were tested: cyclamates, saccharin, and a metabolite of cyclamates) resulted in the banning of just one of those chemicals. Presumably it was because the currently popular table sweeteners and solutions used to artificially sweeten soft drinks and diet products had a 10:1 cyclamate/saccharin ratio, so it was assumed that cyclamates were "more guilty."

Although it escaped a ban in 1969, the saccharin drama began to unfold that very year. First, it was obvious that the elimination of cyclamates meant that the consumption of the only remaining artificial sweetener would soar. Second, the possible coconspirator role of saccharin in the "cyclamania" incident was never forgotten by those who, for whatever reason, had lingering doubts about saccharin's safety.

After 1970, new and occasionally unsettling data started to appear. One study, conducted by the Wisconsin Alumni Research Foundation (WARF), noted that some rats developed bladder tumors when their diet consisted of 5 percent saccharin (a huge percentage of anyone's or anything's diet). Another, conducted by the FDA, found tumorous masses in 3 out of 672 rats fed various amounts of the sweet substance. At least thirty other laboratory studies conducted after 1970 found no significant increase in bladder tumors in mice, but it was the WARF and FDA studies that made the headlines.

It didn't take long for the FDA to feel the pressure of those waving the Delaney flag, and in 1972 the agency removed saccharin from the GRAS list, issuing an order in the Federal Register which placed restrictions on its use. All products containing saccharin then were required to carry a packaging disclaimer stating that it was a "nonnutritive artificial sweetener for persons who must restrict their intake of ordinary sweets." At the same time it was recommended that adults use no more than one gram a day—that is, limit consumption to the equivalent of about seven 12-ounce bottles of diet soda.

And the studies went on. In the meantime, while toxicologists around the world were stuffing laboratory animals with saccharin and looking for tumors, epidemiologists, those medical detectives who analyze human disease patterns, were following some other leads that might shed light on saccharin as a cause of disease. Specifically, they were asking two questions: First, if saccharin is a cancer-causing agent, what type of cancer would it cause and how might the use of the sweetener be reflected in modern-day cancer trends? The answer here was fairly clear (and comforting). If it were to have a cancer-causing effect, the sweetener would probably have as its target such organs as the stomach, bladder, or pancreas—as opposed, for example, to the lung or breast. A look at cancer trends in this country confirmed that only one form of cancer death had increased significantly since 1945—lung cancer, the overwhelming majority of cases of which are attributable to increased cigarette smoking after World War I. Clearly then, saccharin was not responsible for any detectable rise in human cancer deaths.

Second, and even more to the point, was the question: Is there any direct evidence that saccharin consumption increases the probability of cancer development in humans? Modern-day medical ethics forbids the type of human experimentation which was carried out during Dr. Wiley's "poison squad" days back at the turn of the century, but there is such a thing as a "natural experiment"; that is, one where you can glean information from circumstances where specific groups of people are exposed, for nonexperimental reasons, to a chemical or condition for long periods of time. Saccharin proved to be an ideal substance for such a "natural experiment," as diabetics around the world had been using the sweetener since the turn of the century.

A close look at thousands of individuals, some of whom had used the sweetener for twenty-five years or longer, and most all of whom consumed saccharin at a rate ten times that of nondiabetics, found that not only was the cancer death rate among high-level saccharin users not higher but it was actually lower than that of the general population. (The fact that it was lower is explained by the fact that diabetics are much less likely to smoke cigarettes than are nondiabetics. Some 80 percent of all lung cancer deaths and some 30 percent of all bladder cancer deaths are cigarette-induced; in the latter case, the bladder is involved because the body makes a valiant attempt to excrete the tobacco carcinogens.)

In early 1975, the National Academy of Science's National Research Council completed a new study for the FDA—"Safety of Saccharin and Sodium Saccharin in the Human Diet"—and concluded that "on the basis of available information, the present and future usage of saccharin in the United States does not pose a hazard." The gist of the Academy's report was that there was no reason to suspect that saccharin caused cancer in animals (the Academy felt the highly publicized FDA and WARF studies were poorly done and what they did find was not terribly alarming). And there was epidemiological evidence that saccharin did *not* have a carcinogenic effect in man. Nevertheless, it was recommended that animal studies continue in order to resolve all possible doubts. Additionally, the NAS recommended that those human studies of diabetics (mentioned above) be conducted.

Further studies of saccharin began. But, because there was no reason to do otherwise, the FDA on January 7, 1977 granted an "extension of the saccharin regulation". In other words, we were told we could go on eating and drinking it. At that time the Agency noted that a Canadian study was in process and that "about a year from now" data would be compiled and evaluated.

It was rather surprising, then, that two months later, in early March of 1977, the great saccharin controversy broke. Preliminary results of this Canadian study were announced. The findings showed that of 100 rats fed huge amounts of saccharin (5 percent of their total diet) 3 developed bladder tumors; of a group of 100 rats exposed to the sweetener at these doses while they were in their mothers' uteri and exposed throughout their own entire lifetimes, 14 developed bladder tumors. On the basis of these preliminary findings, derived from a somewhat unusual study protocol (exposing animals to "double jeopardy," before and after birth, is not a routine way of evaluating chemical safety. We do not know, for instance, how animals fed salt, sugar, or mustard would have reacted in the same circumstances), the Canadian government banned saccharin on March 9. The same day the American FDA followed suit, noting that under the rule of the Delaney Clause, it had no choice. The implications for Americans were more serious than they were for Canadians in that cyclamates are routinely available on an over-the-counter-drug basis in Canada, but are not available in any form here.

A few weeks later, the FDA somewhat modified the ban by proposing that saccharin be allowed as an over-the-counter drug, for use as a tabletop sweetener (if it could meet the requirements as a drug).

But then a number of weeks after that, the saccharin saga took another twist: the results of a second Canadian study were made available to the press, this time noting a cancer-causing effect of saccharin in human beings. For many people—including Food and Drug Administration Commissioner Dr. Donald Kennedy, this second set of Canadian findings was enough to confirm their earlier impression that saccharin should be banned as a food additive. As Commissioner Kennedy put it, "the new and direct evidence of human risk from saccharin suggested by the Canadian study . . . raises serious questions about the wisdom of our present proposal to consider the continued approval of saccharin for drug use."

But after examining the report of this second Canadian study, one might not find the results as alarming as Commissioner Kennedy's comments might suggest. The study, which was eventually published in the British medical journal, *The Lancet,* was based on a comparison of 632 persons with bladder cancer (480 males, 152 females) and a corresponding number of individuals without bladder cancer. The results showed a bladder cancer risk ratio of 1.6 for users of artificial sweeteners (principally saccharin) versus nonusers. This means that there is an estimated 60 percent increase in the risk of bladder cancer associated with the use of artificial sweeteners in males.

There are three reasons why we urge caution in interpreting

these results as evidence of the human "cancer causing effect" of saccharin. First, a number of different factors are known to be involved in the causation of human bladder cancer, specifically, cigarette smoking and certain occupational exposures. We are not convinced after reading the Canadian report that these factors were adequately taken into account, that is part of the difference noted may have been the result not of saccharin use, but of cigarette smoking, occupational chemicals or some other factor.

Second, while much was made in the press over the 60 percent increase in bladder cancer risk in males, it was only infrequently mentioned that this Canadian study showed a *decreased* risk in bladder cancer (40 percent) for females. This, we feel, is a highly implausible result, one which casts doubt on the overall conclusions of the study, as there is no example that we know of where a chemical which causes cancer in humans of one sex does not have a similar effect on the other sex.

Third, the study is not consistent with other epidemiological studies undertaken by prominent scientists from around the world. All of the previous epidemiology, which included at least eight studies involving 60,000 people, showed no adverse effects from saccharin use. For example, one study of over 18,000 bladder cancer patients compared with 19,000 non-affected individuals (a study which involved more than 30 times as many individuals as the Canadian research) found no "evidence of an increased risk of bladder cancer in diabetics, some of whom must have consumed above average amounts of saccharin for more than 20 years". In another study performed at Johns Hopkins, cyclamate-saccharin consumption patterns of 209 bladder cancer patients were compared to a similar number of individuals without the disease. No evidence of a relationship between saccharin ingestion and bladder cancer was found. And in the most recently completed study, Dr. Ernst Wynder of the American Health Foundation found no relationship between bladder cancer and saccharin consumption among 574 male and 158 female bladder cancer patients and a similar number of matched controls.

The Calorie Control Council, an Atlanta-based international association of leading manufacturers and suppliers of calorie control and dietetic food and beverage products, called the original banning an "example of colossal government overregulation in disregard of science and the needs and wants of the consumer." The Council immediately took out a two-page ad in the Sunday *New York Times* and other papers encouraging consumers to express their outrage to their Congressional representatives. Within forty-eight hours of the announcement of the intended ban, grocery-store shelves were stripped of Sweet 'n' Low and other tabletop sweeteners, and supplies of diet soft drinks had dwindled considerably. (One could not help note the irony of the situation: the FDA had issued a warning to the public of a possible cancer threat and shoppers were literally fighting to get this allegedly harmful product. If the FDA had made a similar announcement, say, about the possible presence of botulism toxin in mushrooms, it is difficult to imagine a similar type of buying stampede.)

Professional groups applied pressure of their own: The American Diabetes Association urged the government to "reexamine its approach to announcing concern and actions to the American people." Newspapers around the country issued irate editorials, one in *The New York Times* demanding that the Delaney Clause, the immediate cause of the saccharin ban, be modified or updated. Of all the major newspapers, only the *Washington Post* supported the banning of the sweetener.

But probably the most interesting and potentially significant reactions occurred on Capitol Hill. Representative James G. Martin (R./N.C., who holds a Ph.D in organic chemistry) requested a stay of execution until the saccharin matter could be reviewed by Congress. Numerous other bills called for either giving the FDA greater discretion in the control of food additives—banning food additives only when they were found to induce cancer when ingested in amounts reasonably anticipated to be consumed by man—or simply called for a general postponement of the saccharin ban. A bill introduced by Representative Jacobs (D.-Ind.), H.R. 4943, entitled "The Un-Crazying of Federal Regulations Act of 1977," included a provision for a warning label on saccharin containers: "Warning: The Canadians have determined that saccharin is dangerous to your rat's health."

At the time of this writing, the future of saccharin—and whether the American public will accept the FDA compromise which would ban its use in soft drinks and other diet products but allow it as a tabletop sweetener if it could be shown that saccharin met the criteria of an "effective drug"—is unclear. What is clear, however, is that, unfortunately, many of the voices raised in protest of the ban served only to confuse an already complex issue. For example, reliance on the following common arguments distracted from the main point.

1. *"But diabetics need it . . . you shouldn't ban it. . . ."*

While this is true, it is a somewhat misleading argument. Certainly artificial sweeteners are a valuable aid to the country's 10 million diabetics and the people should not be deprived of them. But that goal could be accomplished by making saccharin a drug—prescription or otherwise—freely available only to those with a medical need. Indeed, this is what the FDA proposed. This argument obscures the broader issue that for many Americans, saccharin is desirable for other than strict medical reasons, and that by banning the substance, the individual's rights are being compromised.

2. *"Sugar is the real villain . . . given that sugar consumption will increase, the banning of saccharin will cause much greater hazard to human health than would allowing it to stay."*

A misleading, unconstructive charge. Despite the popular assumptions to the contrary, sugar as used in the American diet is not a cause of major systemic disease. There is no evidence that it induces or predisposes toward the development of diabetes (although certainly uncontrolled ingestion of sugar and other carbohydrates can exacerbate this condition). The key factor in predisposition to diabetes is obesity, not sugar consumption. There is no scientific evidence that sugar increases the likelihood of heart disease, as has so often been contended in the popular press. And given that obesity is a condition induced by too many calories eaten and too few expended, it is simplistic and inaccurate to conclude that "sugar makes you fat" and that artificially sweetened products will keep you thin. Of course, sugar is a source of calories, and if one consumes a great deal of sweets one will put on weight. Yet, curiously, numerous studies have concluded that obese individuals are less likely than nonobese individuals to use moderate or large amounts of sugar, instead they tend to get their calories from other sources, like fats and alcohol.

3. *"It's like a human drinking 1,200 bottles of diet soda a day. Anything at that dose could cause cancer. We shouldn't ban something on the basis of irrelevant experiments like that."*

Again, we have here a defense which could be legitimately challenged both by scientists and nonscientists. The fact is that animal experiments *are* useful in gathering information on food and drug and other chemical safety. And everything does *not* cause cancer. Since we can't directly experiment on humans, the laboratory species are about all we have. And in doing such tests scientists *must* use large quantities of the substance being tested, because (among other reasons) the animals have such a short lifetime and if disease is to be induced, it must be induced quickly.

The issue in the saccharin case, and other cases where the Delaney Clause has been applied, is not the fact that large quantities were being used but rather that there was no relationship between the amount of saccharin consumed by the animals and the appearance of tumors, that the positive results were limited to one type of animal—and that despite the lack of such a relationship, a ban was called for anyway.

If the Canadian saccharin study—or another study before or after it—showed a clear dose response, that is, that the rats drinking the equivalent of 200, 400, 600, 800, 1,200 bottles of soda a day developed an increasing number of tumors—*and* if this finding was confirmed in other species—say, a guinea pig, dog or monkey, the results would be worth noting and a call for a ban on saccharin would have much more justification.

4. *"Well, we might lose saccharin, but there will be another artificial sweetener on the horizon soon."*

This argument reflects undue optimism, both in terms of research goals and regulatory reform. There is *no* artificial sweetener likely to be approved for general use immediately. Aspartame, originally approved by the FDA three years ago, never made it to the market because of some isolated reports about adverse health effects on monkeys, and the fact that its manufacturer, G. D. Searle, was facing charges of mishandling animal experiments and falsifying data. Even if it did get approval within a year or two, it is nowhere near as flexible as saccharin, and would not gain approval for use in soft drinks or bakery products. Xylitol, a sweetener made chiefly from birchwood, is still being tested; it has the disadvantage of having a diuretic effect in large amounts, a characteristic which would make it unacceptable for soft drinks. Neohesperidine dihydrochalcone, an extract of discarded orange and grapefruit peels, which has received a great deal of attention, is many years away from being introduced. Cyclamates, banned in 1969, are still caught in a bitter legal controversy; the mechanism for lifting a ban on a food additive is yet to be worked out.

Even if one or more of these sweeteners entered the market within a year or so, they would still be subject to our current laws, and someone, somewhere would eventually show that sweet-tooth rodents developed tumors.

Additionally, common sense makes it questionable to introduce a new and, relatively speaking, untested sweetener to replace one which has been used for over eighty years with no indication of causing harm to human health.

5. *"Just label saccharin products 'This product may be harmful to your health.' Then people can decide for themselves."*

This is an unacceptable and unrealistic alternative. Indeed, it might do more harm than good in that it would confuse people. The warning label on saccharin would be equated with the warning label on cigarettes, although the evidence indicting these two products as a health risk are miles apart, one being a hypothetical risk, one being a real one. Furthermore, to be consistent, *everything* in the store would have to be labeled. Yogurt, too. Even though it's "natural," it has caused cataracts in mice when fed at very high doses (an observation confirmed by a number of laboratory experiments).

These five smoke screens, set up after the FDA announcement by a variety of well-meaning individuals, obscured the main point: we *need* rational, politically neutral, scientifically based laws, ones *which take into account consumers wants and needs,* to ensure the safety and availability of a wide variety of drugs and foods. We do need a federal regulatory system to ensure that environmental chemicals—including additives, pesticides, drugs, and those used in industrial plants—are, by current standards, safe. There are legitimate instances in which government agencies have acted decisively and correctly. For example, the FDA has refused to approve a preparation known as laetrile, which has been repeatedly shown to be ineffective in the prevention or treatment of cancer. The National Institute for Occupational Safety and Health and other related Federal groups have set strict standards to control worker exposure to such cancer-causing chemicals as vinyl chloride and asbestos.

What we do *not* need in the field of food and drug regulation is a law so arbitrary that it precludes choices and creates a situation in which the majority opinion is overruled by a minority report or view. This majority opinion may be a scientifically based one which notes that an additive is needed to protect health or increase food supply. Or it can be a *consumer* majority opinion based on the fact that an additive—in this case, the sweetener saccharin—*adds enjoyment to life and allows a choice in decisions about food and beverages.*

How could we resolve the Delaney dilemma and keep saccharin-sweetened soft drinks and products with other useful food additives on the shelves? Probably the most effective and reasonable approach would be to delete the Delaney Clause from the lawbooks. Its forty-seven words are unnecessary and redundant. The FDA already has the legal power to regulate the safety of ingested products. (More detailed comments on the Delaney Clause will be made in Chapter 14.)

But, the political reality, given the widespread concern about cancer causation and the possible link with chemicals in food, is that the immediate excision of the Delaney Clause is not a likely event. At the time of this writing, it seems more probable that a sidestepping approach will be taken in an effort limited to the salvation of saccharin: the Canadian study could be labeled "inappropriate" (critiques of the report have already been issued by the Calorie Control Council and other such groups). If the test is declared inappropriate, the conditions of the Delaney Clause would not have been met and thus we could go on gulping diet soda. Or the Delaney Clause could be amended in a way that would permit the FDA to make a decision on sweeteners on the basis of comparative risks—that is, choosing among saccharin, cyclamates, and aspartame as to the safest artificial sweetener.

Or, taking a more general (if only interim) tack, Congress could amalgamate the various "modify Delaney bills" before it now, and decide to add a phrase at the end of the Clause allowing an animal carcinogen or suspected animal carcinogen in the food supply if there were a greater medical, social, or psychological risk from banning it.

The immediate future of our food laws in general and saccharin in particular, are at this point unclear. But what is clear is that because of the saccharin flap, the Delaney Clause may have been dealt a mortal wound, one which may well accelerate our entrance into an age of new and more reasonable approaches to evaluating the chemicals in our lives.

12

STRESS

"Let me speak to you regarding the things of which you must beware. To get angry and shout at times pleases me, for this will keep up your natural heat; but what displeases me is your being grieved and taking all matters to heart. For it is this, as the whole physic teaches which destroys our body more than any other cause."

Dr. Maestro Lorenzo Sassoli,
in a letter written to a patient in 1402

A MIND-BODY LINK?

Mrs. Emerson, upon the Death of her Daughter, underwent great Affliction, and perceived her Breast to swell, which soon after grew painful; at last broke out in a most inverterate Cancer, which consumed a great Part of it in a short Time. She had always enjoy'd a perfect state of health.

The Wife of a Mate of a Ship (who was taken some Time ago by the French, and put in Prison) was thereby so much affected, that her breast began to swell, and soon after broke out in a desperate cancer which had proceeded so far that I could not undertake her case. She never before had any complaint in her breast.

During the 18th and 19th centuries, there were a number of reports like the above made by physicians and nonphysicians alike, the suggestion being that grief, or some other form of life stress, can bring about cancer, or as the renowned physician Sir James Paget wrote, "The cases are frequent in which deep anxiety, deferred hope and disappointment are quickly followed by the growth or increase of cancer. . . ."

The idea is still very much with us today, and indeed has taken on a broader scope: A number of researchers have suggested that both stress and the way we handle it can influence the odds on developing many diseases, including cancer.

What Is Stress?

Dr. Hans Selye has defined stress as "the nonspecific response of the body to any demand upon it." It is not simple nervous tension nor is it something that we can escape entirely. We are under physiological stress even when we are fully relaxed and asleep. The only real freedom from stress is death.

But the type of stress that we are interested in here is the variety which goes beyond the everyday expected type: conflicts with your spouse, boss, or fellow workers; extreme grief over the illness or death of a close friend or relative; a major economic loss, a drastic change in lifestyle. Does this type of stress have any effect on disease patterns?

Stress and Animals

Animal experiments indicate that stress does have an important biological effect, leaving an animal disease-prone. Dr. Selye has shown in numerous laboratory experiments that animals under stress (whether it is extreme cold, frustration, screaming sirens nearby) suffer "internal wreckage," blood pressure soars, autopsies show enlargement of the adrenal glands, shrunken thymus, and peptic ulcers.

Some recent demonstrations conducted by Dr. Vernon Riley and his colleagues, Dr. Darrel Spackman and George Santisteban at the Pacific Northwest Research Foundation at the Fred Hutchinson Cancer Research Center in Seattle, have demonstrated that stress factors in mice bring about physiological changes which apparently affect their susceptibility to cancer. In one experiment recently reported in *Science,* he selected a group of mice (C 3H) which is usually highly cancer-prone. Indeed, under most conditions 80 to 100 percent of these animals develop breast tumors within eight to eighteen months after birth. But when Dr. Riley put these mice behind a protective barrier, keeping them free of the normal laboratory noise and other commotion which might generate anxiety and stress, only 7 percent developed cancer after fourteen months. Dr. Riley further showed that even mild anxiety stress, say rotating mice slowly on a turntable for a few minutes out of each hour, will increase their probability of developing malignancies.

The stress the animals experience evidently brings about significant changes in hormones which interfere with the animal's defense system against cancer. For instance, Dr. Riley has been able to demonstrate that the adrenal glands of stressed animals are spurred into action, and the animals' blood levels of corticosterone, the hormone equivalent to cortisol in human beings, increase significantly. Excess levels of this hormone, in turn, damage important elements of the defense apparatus (thymus and T cells), which leaves the animal vulnerable to cancer cells, viruses, and other disease processes. Interestingly, "artificial stress"—and a related higher probability of cancer—can be *induced* in animals by injecting them with that chemical sign of stress—corticosterone.

Are there any implications in this research for humans? Now, the only answer to that question is, "Maybe."

If we are in good health, our "cancer surveillance" system is operating effectively. Under one theory we encounter cancer-causing agents every day, yet we are not affected by them because our immune system rejects them before they can begin the cancer growth process.

If we follow the same stress-response pattern of animals a significant and /or prolonged stress may interfere with that "surveillance" system. Specifically, when we encounter stressful events—be it extreme fear, strong emotions, anger, depression—a chain of biological events is set off. Our adrenal and pituitary glands produce ACTH, cortisone, and other hormones which stimulate protective body reactions. *Some* of these stress-induced chemical changes probably cause no ill effects—the body still goes on fighting off carcinogens. But if the system gets overloaded there may be serious trouble. Indeed, excessive amounts of those perfectly natural physiological changes which accompany stress may damage our immunologic apparatus to the extent that we are left vulnerable, even if for a short period of time. As Dr. Riley emphasizes, "Anything that affects the immune system has the potential to affect many disease processes, including cancer. With this breakdown in immune responses—even if temporary—the cancer-causing agent has a chance to get its foot in the door—and it's on its way."

Evidence in Humans?

William A. Greene, a psychiatrist at the University of Rochester, studied the life history of three sets of twins. One twin out of each set developed leukemia. He found that the twin who developed leukemia had experienced a psychological upheaval right before the onset of the disease. The other twin had not. Dr. Greene concluded that psychological trauma might well be a precipitating factor in cancer—even stronger than genetic predisposition.

Dr. H. J. F. Baltrusch, a researcher from the International Psychosomatic and Cross-Cultural Leukemic Project in West Germany, agrees. He reported to the Third International Symposium on Detection and Prevention of Cancer that, having studied more than eight thousand patients with different types of cancerous lesions, "In the majority of patients clinical manifestations of malignancy occurred during a period of severe and intensive life stress involving frequently loss, separation and other bereavements."

Is There a "Cancer-Prone" Personality?

Not only is it suggested that severe life stress may be important in bringing about or promoting cancer, but some have hypothesized that the way we handle that stress might also be a key.

During the period 1946 to 1964, Dr. Caroline B. Thomas collected physical and psychological profiles of 1,337 medical students at Johns Hopkins. She kept track of them by means of yearly questionnaires, noting the cause of death if it occurred. Dr. Thomas found that cancers tended to develop in people who were generally quiet, nonaggressive, and emotionally contained. These were generally "low gear" patients, seldom prone to outbursts of emotions.

Dr. Rene C. Mastrovito, a psychiatrist from the Department of Neurology at Memorial Sloan-Kettering Cancer Center in New York, recently told the International Symposium that he had additional evidence to support the existence of a "cancer-prone" personality. He and his associates studied women who were admitted to the hospital for suspected or confirmed cancer of the ovary, uterus, cervix and vagina, and compared these to women who had no suspected cancer (the study was done before the cancer diagnosis was made, so the stress which would accompany knowledge of the disease was not present). Dr. Mastrovito found that women who were diagnosed as having cancer were much more conforming, less adventurous, assertive, competitive, and spontaneous than were those women in the noncancer group. Dr. Mastrovito's observations were immediately bolstered by those of Dr. S. Greer from King's College Hospital in London in that breast cancer patients there demonstrated "an abnormal release of emotions"—particularly extreme suppression of anger. In other words, their reaction to stress was denial—a bottling up of feelings.

Drs. Claus and Marjorie Bahnson, a husband-wife psychology team at the Eastern Pennsylvania Psychiatric Institute, have now developed a questionnaire which covers topics such as loss and reactions to loss of close relatives by death, stress, and recent life changes, personality characteristics and means of handling stress. They feel this research-diagnostic tool catches potential cancer victims early, while effective treatment is still available and practical.

STRESS, CANCER, AND YOU

Both the animal experiments and human observations about the possible role of stress in predisposing one to cancer are fascinating and worthy of further study. The implications that the body's immune system might be adversely affected could, in the future, prove to be a vital lead in cancer research. Presumably if solid evidence were ever gathered about environmentally induced shifts in our body's defense system, a type of blocking agent which could keep the body on an even-hormonal keel despite the aggravating external events could prove to be a lifesaver.

But despite the appeal that this "mind-body" link might have, the role of stress in the causation of human cancer is, at best, a hypothetical one. The concept of a "psychological upheaval" appearing before the onset of disease is a difficult one to measure, very much influenced by the patient's recall, which could be colored by his or her traumatic experience. Observations that cancer patients have often experienced severe personal losses just prior to their disease overlook the fact that cancer is a disease that strikes late in life; at a time when one's friends, spouse, and many close relatives are subject to sudden death. The average age of widowhood is fifty-seven or fifty-eight in the United States. The late fifties are also a prime time for the development of breast cancer. Whether these two events have anything to do with each other is now just a matter of speculation.

Right now we have no information which would lead us to conclude that any of the major forms of cancer in the United States are caused, even indirectly, by stressful conditions or a personality that "keeps things inside."

13

AIR POLLUTION

"Air pollution is turning Mother Nature
prematurely gray."

Irv Kupcinet

"I live in Manhattan. The air is so bad there, it's like smoking two packs a day. That pollution is bound to give you lung cancer."

Our lungs are our main contact with the outside world. We breathe about twenty times every minute, inhaling and exhaling a pint of air with each breath. The air in many of our cities is far from acceptable, very often containing various amounts of substances known to cause cancer in experiment animals. Of particular concern is the presence of some polycyclic aromatic hydrocarbons (PAH's), the most easily detectable of which is benzo(a)pyrene (BP).

The questions here are: Are carcinogens present in the air in sufficient quantity to cause human cancer? As the oft-heard statement above suggests, does breathing polluted city air pose the same or similar risk of lung cancer as does cigarette smoking?

CITIES, POLLUTION AND CANCER

Let's for a moment assume that air pollution does play at least some role in cancer causation in this country. After all, it is not inconsistent with our knowledge about cancer causation that inhaling a carcinogenic substance might put us at risk. For instance, we've already seen that the inhalation of asbestos and various ores in industrial situations increases the odds on those workers' chances of developing lung cancer. Simply because polluted air comes in frequent contact with our lungs, as opposed to other parts of our body, we might assume that the cancer effect, if it is to occur, would be focused on those organs. This is not to exclude the possibility that if air pollution does have a carcinogenic effect, it could exert it on a number of internal organs. But for the sake of simplifying the discussion, let's stick with the lungs.

If air pollution is involved as a causative factor in lung cancer, then we should expect some consistent findings. First, lung cancer rates should have increased some twenty to thirty years after the air became increasingly polluted in this country. Second, countries with low levels of air pollution should have relatively low rates of lung cancer mortality. Third, urban areas should have higher lung cancer mortality than nonurban areas.

Trends

Lung cancer was a very rare disease early in this century. It did not begin to become a significant cause of death until 1925. But pollution from coal smoke has been with us for at least one hundred years before that.

But, some have argued, the intensity of the pollution did not become great until after 1925. So perhaps air pollution did play a role in the soaring United States lung cancer death rate.

There is, however, a serious flaw in that argument: the upward rise in lung cancer has not affected both men and women equally. Presumably, if air pollution were involved in the causation of this disease, since both males and females were breathing the same air, both should have been equally affected.

Of course, the more obvious explanation here is that the surge in the male lung cancer rate is the result of males being exposed to a factor, namely cigarette smoking, much more frequently than were women.

Countries

As in the United States, the death rate from cancer of the lung is a major cause of mortality in many westernized countries, including Australia, Austria, Switzerland, and Iceland, countries one does not generally associate with high levels of air pollution.

Urban versus Rural

Lung cancer does occur more often in cities than it does in the rural portions of the country. But in addition to the air being different in these two types of localities, the people and other community characteristics are different. Of minor, although not insignificant, importance, is that cities have more facilities for diagnosing lung cancer. Of somewhat more significance is that more city dwellers may have in the past had some type of occupational exposure which predisposed them to developing lung cancer. Of major importance is that people living in cities, whether because of socioeconomic class differences (a greater portion of lower and middle socioeconomic-class individuals in this country smoke cigarettes than do those in the upper middle and upper classes, and the population of our cities overrepresents lower socioeconomic people) or because of "personality factors" (a fast pace of life, nervousness, pressurized working conditions), *city dwellers smoke cigarettes more often than do non-city-dwellers.*

Studies which have taken into account the proportion of the population that smokes cigarettes have found that the differences in mortality from lung cancer between cities and rural areas has been considerably diminished. Presumably, if the type of smoking habits—amount smoked, use of filters and nonfilters, age at which smoking began, degree of inhalation—were taken into account, the differences here would disappear completely.

Cigarettes and Polluted Air

Drs. Ernst Wynder and Dietrich Hoffman of the American Health Foundation have pointed out that if you lived for twenty-four hours a day in Herald Square, New York City—and very few of us do—you would be inhaling, in terms of carcinogens, the equivalent of about four and a half cigarettes a day.

But the comparison here is not fully valid because there are major differences in the way the inhalation occurs in breathing air and sucking in tobacco smoke.

When you breathe, it is generally done through your nose. You benefit from the complex natural defense system of your respiratory tract. A significant number of the contaminants in air are filtered out before they ever get to your lungs.

Mother Nature evidently did not anticipate that 20th century man would be foolish enough to inhale hot air, with a heavy concentration of carcinogens, *directly* into his lungs. Drs. Hoffman and Wynder further note that "the cigarette smoker who inhales through his mouth ingests up to five billion particles per cubic centimeter of smoke. The respiratory mechanism is hardly capable of adequate removal of such a dense aerosol. By breathing even heavily polluted air through his nose, a man will inhale a maximum of 100,000 particles per cubic centimeter of air." Again, in this latter case, the filtering system goes to work, and does a very efficient job.

A smoker of twenty cigarettes per day is likely to inhale more than 500 milligrams of concentrated tar, almost all of which bypasses the upper respiratory tract, and goes directly to the lungs.

This dismissal of air pollution as a known cancer risk does *not* mean that in the future—with increasing amounts of carcinogens in our air—it could never be a threat. But in terms of our own attempts to avoid cancer in the late 1970s, air pollution should not be one of our major concerns.[1]

Recent reports about the cancer mortality rate in the highly industrialized state of New Jersey may appear to contradict this general conclusion that pollution is not a factor in cancer etiology. Thus a word about the New Jersey situation is in order.

1. The position taken here is that polluted air is a hypothetical, not an established cause of human cancer. In fairness, however, it should be noted, that there is some slight disagreement among scientists on this subject. A recent report of a research team from the Departments of Community Medicine and Pathology at the University of Southern California School of Medicine concluded that air pollution had a "small, but not negligible" effect on cancer risk.

A National Cancer Institute county by county study of cancer deaths in the United States between 1950 and 1969 placed this state in the unenviable position of being "number one" in cancer mortality. There is no doubt that the strikingly high cancer of the bladder death rate is related to the industrial use of certain chemicals, such as beta napthalamine, which was used in the manufacture of dyes during the 1950s. At the same time, New Jersey had one of the greatest concentration of other chemical plants in the world (and still does). One chemical known to induce human cancer—vinyl chloride—is manufactured in fifty-eight plants in the United States, five of which are in New Jersey.

But the majority of excessive cancer mortality in New Jersey cannot be explained by industrial exposures. New Jersey ranks first for ovarian cancers among white women and rectal cancers for both white and black women and ranks third and fourth for breast cancer (white and nonwhite women respectively). None of these cancers have ever been linked with industrial exposure. In lung cancer, New Jersey placed about fourth in the nation but, as has been previously mentioned in this chapter and elsewhere in this book, lung cancer mortality is largely explained by cigarette smoking.

A research team from the Department of Preventive Medicine and Community Health at New Jersey Medical School and the Cancer Institute of New Jersey concluded, after analyzing the figures, that only about seven hundred or 5 percent of the estimated 1976 cancer deaths in that state can be attributed to industrial exposure. What is critical to keep in mind here is that the 'industrial exposure" refers not to the general population, but to workers who ten, fifteen, twenty, or more years ago were exposed to industrial carcinogens.

AN AIR POLLUTION THREAT?

There is no doubt that our air now contains things that should not be there. These contaminants do play a role in diseases, such as chronic bronchitis, emphysema, and asthma, and the chaos which has followed the major air inversions of the past forty years has shown that. We should do everything technologically feasible to make our air pure.

For example, on Friday, December 5, 1952, the air of London, England, became a deadly menace. A prolonged temperature inversion coupled with an anticyclonic high-pressure system held the city's air close to the ground, prevented winds from dispersing pollutants and forced the city's routine air pollutant emissions to accumulate heavily at ground level. Following five days of virtually unbreatheable air, four thousand more deaths than normal were recorded, 84 percent of them among people with preexisting heart and lung diseases. A similar type of inversion occurred in Donora, Pennsylvania in 1948.

Our conclusion here is not "everything is okay with the air." But our interest in this book is exclusively on cancer threats. In classifying air pollution as a "hypothetical" cancer risk, we are relying on the research of a wide number of scientists. The Royal College of Physicians in 1970, after throughly examining the possible role of air pollution in human carcinomas, concluded "the study of time trends on the death rate due to lung cancer in urban areas demonstrated the overwhelming effect of cigarette smoking on the distribution of disease." Drs. Wynder and Hoffman agree, noting that "on the basis of data accumulated in the United States, we cannot conclude that the incidence of lung cancer is much affected by community air pollution in this country."

Ironically, many people who are worried about the adverse health effects of air pollution overlook the most obvious form that we come in contact with: one cigarette smoker, in a matter of minutes, can fill a closed room with higher concentrations of the carcinogen benzo(a)pyrene than are found in the most polluted city air in the world. If you are worried about the effects of air pollution on your lungs, your best bet would be to ban smoking in your home, and become involved in efforts to isolate smokers in offices and public places.

PART III

14

CANCER:
A PERSPECTIVE

"For man is man and master of his fate."
Lord Alfred Tennyson

We are all understandably worried about cancer. But it appears that in the past, many of us have been worrying about the wrong things. As you saw in the eight chapters on "known causes," we do know a great deal about this disease and what will increase our risks, but ironically, it is the hypothetical risks that get all the attention. The real ones are very infrequently mentioned.

There are two ways you might use the growing information we have about cancer causation: to improve your own (and your family's) personal chances for a long, healthy, and productive life, and to influence our government policies in the area of cancer research and the regulation of cancer-causing agents.

YOUR "WORRY" LIST

There are all types of potential health threats around us. If you had nothing to do all day, you could make a list of them. Maybe Xerox machines cause cancer. Maybe the glue on the back of postage stamps really does contain carcinogenic material. Perhaps getting more than eight hours and less than seven hours sleep, swimming in a pool, chewing on a pencil, watching color TV, or working with scotch tape could increase your risk of cancer. There are limitless possibilities with which you could confuse yourself. But if you are living a busy life, you have but a limited amount of time to dedicate to your personal cancer prevention plan. So the few things that you *do* put on your "worry list" and commit yourself to do something about should be based on the known facts on cancer causation.

What Causes Human Cancer?[a]

CAUSATIVE FACTOR	ESTIMATED PERCENTAGE OF ALL U.S. CANCER DEATHS
Environmental	
Cigarette smoking	30–35%
Imprudent diet	30–35
Occupation	1–2
Background radiation	2–4
Nonenvironmental	
Genetic	4–5
Total, Environmental and Nonenvironmental	67–81
Unaccounted for	19–33

[a] Excluding superficial skin cancer. There are many estimates on the percentage of American cancer deaths attributable to various causes. This chart represents the average figures suggested by various scientists from the National Cancer Institute, American Cancer Society and elsewhere. These are estimates, not official figures.

There are many different estimates about what percentage of cancer is caused by this or that, but this summary table should help you when you sit down to determine what should be the top two items on your worry list.

Presumably some of the "unaccounted" causes include virally induced cancers, like cancer of the cervix, and other cases related to excessive alcohol use, medical uses of radiation, and most important, a general body deterioration which accompanies aging and may account for some "spontaneous" cancer deaths.

Given that the first two environmental causes, cigarette smoking and imprudent diet account for two-thirds to three-quarters of all cancer deaths, it is clear what the first two factors on your worry list should be. (The appendixes which follow offer some practical advice in these areas.)

Dr. Marvin A. Schneiderman of the National Cancer Institute has observed that the most effective public health measures are always those which people do not have to do for themselves. For instance, when water supplies were treated with chlorine, gastrointestinal-tract diseases declined precipitously. All the individual had to do was to pay a relatively small amount of community tax for this service. The second most effective public health measure is the type that people have to do only a few times in a lifetime—for instance, get a tetanus shot. There's really not too much effort there. The least effective public health measure is the type that individuals have to do themselves on a regular basis. It is this third, difficult category that we are dealing with here in our effort to avoid cancer.

If you are to be successful in minimizing your risks of cancer, you must, on your own initiative, take preventive steps outlined in Chapters 3 through 10. *If you, for reason of lack of motivation or because you think you are "too old to change," do not pattern your life-style in the ways recommended in this book, then at least be sure that your children and grandchildren do!*

CANCER AND PUBLIC POLICY

This book has been relatively limited in scope in that it has concentrated on the ways you, right now, can change your life in a way that will help you avoid cancer. But we should end on a broader note.

If we are going to further increase our knowledge about this disease, possibly even developing new protective measures, a preventive vaccine, or a cure, we must both redirect our priorities in the area of cancer research *and* reevaluate our current attitudes about identifying possible causes of human cancer.

The Delaney Clause

High on our list of "things to do" to influence cancer research policy should be efforts to modernize the legislation which governs both additives, pesticides, drugs—and known human carcinogens.

In 1958, Congress approved the Delaney Clause,[1] requiring that an additive or pesticide be banned if it was shown to cause cancer in any experiment in any animal. This piece of legislation has probably caused more confusion in the area of cancer research than any other law, and has only served to call repeated attention to hypothetical cancer risks like cyclamates and red dye #2, while distracting people from the things they should be concerned about. The statute is a medical and legal tragedy, an example of how the real spirit of law can be thwarted by personal politics and unrestrained advocacy. The Clause has good intentions—after all, no American in his right mind would want to add cancer-causing chemicals to our food supply. Indeed, because of its underlying good intentions, the Clause has great appeal to common sense and emotions of the average person. But in practical terms—and in dealing with the realities of what causes human cancer—the Delaney Clause is at best scientifically naïve, and at worst, dangerously misleading. It is a law based on a highly emotionally charged fear of a devastating disease—cancer—and it is an underlying cause of another serious and widespread American ailment—cancerphobia.

Because the Clause is such an important factor in directing the course of cancer research and in determining what chemicals should and should not be allowed in our environment—and given that the recently proposed ban on saccharin has engendered a new interest in it—it is worth spending some time here looking at its primary limitations.

First, the Clause is an arbitrary, inflexible statute which requires the banning of a food additive on the basis of one or a limited number of laboratory animal experiments, even though those

1. The Delaney Clause, passed into law in the final hours of debate over the 1958 Food Additive Amendment states that 'no additive shall be deemed to be safe if it is found to induce cancer when ingested by man or animal, or if it is found, after tests which are appropriate for the evaluation of the safety of food additives, to induce cancer in man or animals. . . ."

experiments may contradict the general knowledge about the carcinogenicity of that substance. The lack of discretion in the Delaney Clause contrasts sharply with that afforded in other sections of the food and drug law.

Those defending the position that the addition of the adjective "appropriate" to describe tests capable of invoking the Clause does allow discretion, overlook the fact that the mere existence of the Clause, and the awareness that one set of positive results in a cancer experiment is enough to lead to a banning, creates an atmosphere of fear and urgency where decisions are based not on facts but on what a chemical might possibly do.

Judgments on the relative safety of environmental chemicals are often difficult to make, such decisions involving a series of facts and detailed knowledge of circumstances. Certainly an arbitrary law which says if A happens then B must follow, is a simplistic, carefree basis for regulatory procedure. But it is unrealistic, unsophisticated, and untenable in the world of carcinogenesis, where a multitude of variables may be involved in causation.

Second, the Delaney Clause and related legislative philosophies rely heavily on the assumption that animal experiments are excellent predictors of the cancer-causing potential of a chemical in man. Indeed, proponents of the Clause often point out that all chemicals that cause cancer in man cause cancer in animals, the implicit conclusion being, then, that mice are little men.

While it is true that most—but not all—known human carcinogens are cancer-causing agents in laboratory animals (an exception here would be the known human bladder carcinogen beta-napthylamine which does not have a cancer-causing impact on the bladders of rats or mice), *the opposite is not true*—all animal carcinogens are not known human carcinogens. As is pointed out elsewhere in this book, for example, drugs such as sodium penicillin and phenobarbitol are known animal carcinogens but have no known cancer-causing effect in humans. If the philosophy of the Delaney Clause were applied to the oral contraceptive—which contains a synthetic estrogen—The Pill would never have been approved, because all estrogens, natural, or otherwise, have carcinogenic properties.

There is no doubt that animal experimentation plays a critical role in chemical safety evaluation. Some of the most important medical discoveries had their beginnings in animal experimentation. For instance, our understanding of the biological basis for diabetes began with an experiment where the pancreas was removed from dogs and it was noted that the urine of these animals was unusually sweet, an observation that led to the discovery of insulin's role in this disease. We are not suggesting that we rely solely on evidence of human experience with a substance. Epidemiology does have its limitations, primary among them that it takes five, ten, twenty, or more years for some human carcinogens to make known their deadly characteristics. But we simply cannot be guided by a law which assumes that the laboratory animal is an infallible predictor for man. Animal experiments need to be interpreted, put in proper perspective. Possible individual species or strain susceptibility must be taken into account—as well as other unique circumstances that may have been responsible for whatever positive results may have appeared. For example, morphine in the cat has a directly opposite effect than it has in human beings. Morphine is a very useful sedative, an analgesic drug in man, but when it is given to a cat, the animal becomes restless and belligerent. In the nutritional field, while man and guinea pigs require vitamin C in the diet to protect them from scurvy, the rat does not need an external form of vitamin C. Thus a laboratory experiment using the rat to understand the causation of scurvy would have been futile and misleading.

If a food additive, when ingested by a group of rats, leads to an increased incidence of malignant tumors of the bladder, liver or other organ, the results are worth noting. But that observation is certainly not enough to warrant the condemnation of that additive. Instead, such an observation should stimulate similar tests on other animals. When a series of different tests on different animals are in, the scientific decision-making process could begin—were the results consistent—or somewhat consistent? At the very least, did the chemical have a carcinogenic effect in more than one species? What about a dose-response relationship? Did the incidence of tumors increase as the dosage of the chemical was increased? Does the chemical being evaluated have any characteristics that might lead one to suspect it is carcinogenic? Are there specific factors which promote or inhibit the carcinogenic effect of this substance in a laboratory animal? Is there any human epidemiological evidence available on the substance which would support or fail to support the laboratory findings? Certainly years of safe use by humans (as is the case with saccharin) should carry more weight than one limited animal evaluation. Does the chemical perform an important function? Are there alternatives? The answers to some, if not all, of these questions may provide a basis for sound, scientific decision making. There can be no set rules. The data provided by laboratory experimentation should provide one input into a complex evaluation procedure.

Third, the Delaney Clause (and policies similar to it) are unrealistic and, indeed, anachronistic in that they assume that if large amounts of a substance induce cancer in animals or humans, then even trace amounts—minute quantities—could also be carcinogenic.[2]

This zero tolerance principle is, as is the case with the Clause in general, deceptively simple and emotionally appealing—"Why take the chance?" is the common reasoning. "A little bit of a carcinogen might cause a little bit of cancer, so we should eliminate our exposure to all of it." Such a statement ignores scientific knowledge and capabilities.

All known human cancer-causing agents have some "dose response" curve. Individuals smoking two cigarettes a day for ten or more years show no appreciable increase in mortality from lung cancer. Those smoking ten, fifteen, twenty, thirty or more cigarettes a day show an increasing tendency to die from lung cancer. Individuals who spend a great deal of time in the direct sunlight, particularly if they are fair-skinned, have a high probability of developing skin cancer sometime in their lives. But the fairest of all individuals spending limited time in the sun is highly unlikely to develop a sun-induced skin cancer.

2. This particular problem of the Delaney Clause may become more pronounced as testing techniques become more sophisticated. The so-called Ames test (named after Dr. Bruce N. Ames), which uses colonies of tiny bacteria in small laboratory dishes to test chemicals, instead of time-consuming, expensive animal experiments, and gives reading in two to three days instead of the months and years it takes with more traditional testing, may, because of its high degree of sensitivity, raise more questions about the relevance of "zero tolerance."

Again, proponents of the Clause will claim: "We do not know how to establish with any assurance at all a safe dose in man's food for a cancer-producing substance." That is just another way of saying we can't prove something is safe—which is true. In setting guidelines for chemical exposure—whether in food, the workplace, or elsewhere—what we are looking for are levels which, by all reasonable standards apparently cause no harm.

Related to the problems of the zero tolerance principle, the Delaney Clause is particularly untenable today, given the sophisticated means we have of detecting minute levels of a substance. This limitation of the Clause will become increasingly apparent with the growing sophistication of analytical chemistry. At the time the law was enacted, toxicologists were able to detect adulteration on the order of one part per billion. Today sensitivities are below one part per billion, well on their way to parts per trillion. The problem here was well summarized in a 1973 *New York Times* editorial questioning the original banning of the cattle-growth stimulant DES on the basis of trace amounts of the chemical being found in beef livers: "The Delaney Amendment is an all-or-nothing affair, and presumably would have applied if the analytic equipment had found only one-thousandth of a trillionth part of DES. This sounds more like fanaticism than intelligent public policy. Would not Congress be well advised to consult the scientists on what meaning, if any, the law should give to infinitesimal quantities?"

Fourth, the Clause is inconsistent in that it only applies to food additives. It seems to prefer naturally occurring carcinogens to man-made ones. Thus you have a situation where saccharin, cyclamates, or red dye could be banned as cancer-causing agents—yet it is well known that naturally occurring carcinogens surround us. Safrole, a component of some essential oils and several spices, causes liver tumors in rats, and indeed it was this factor which led to its banning as an artificial food additive. (Aflatoxins, discussed in more detail in Chapter 4, probably the most potent chemical inducers of liver cancer, are molds which grow naturally on such products as peanuts and wheat—but the Delaney Clause is not interested in them.) Estrogens—the source of concern in discussions about the safety of DES in raising cattle—are widely found in nature's own products, wheat, soybeans, green leaves, vegetable oil, all containing far more estrogenic activity than has ever been found in liver from estrogen-treated cattle.

Fifth, the Delaney Clause is blind to the concept of benefit and risk. If nitrites are shown to cause cancer in ducks and removed from the previously sanctioned category so they are vulnerable to the effects of the anticancer Clause, they could be banned even though they are considered essential for protecting us from the deadly botulism toxin.

What is alarming now is that there may be *more* "Delaney-like" forms of legislation introduced in the future if public awareness about the implications are not made known.

For instance, the Environmental Protection Agency has recently drawn up what a British medical journal, *Lancet,* referred to as "Seventeen principles about cancer or something," claiming that a carcinogenic agent is any one that increases any tumor, malignant, or otherwise in animals; that the concept that small doses of a carcinogen may not cause cancer has no practical significance because there is no method for establishing such a level; and that any substances which produce tumors in animals must be considered to be cancer hazards in man. As *Lancet* described it, "The principles vary from the innocuous to the absurd."

If these principles about cancer were to be accepted, cancer evaluation studies would be put in a theoretical straightjacket, and recommendations would be based on a totally inflexible set of regulations, rather than scientific judgment. Again, such rigid rules about what is or is not a carcinogen overlooks the reality that certain basic nutrients, vital drugs, can cause cancer in animals. Guidelines of this nature simply play right into the hands of individuals who are making a career out of chemical witch-hunts.

Distraction and Polarization

Probably the most devastating impact of our current legislative approach to regulating carcinogens is the fact that it acts as a distractionary, divisive factor in the ongoing pursuit of knowledge about what does cause cancer.

With almost weekly reports about allegedly "cancer-causing

agents" in the food supply, cancerphobia in America has intensified and consumers have been distracted from proven human cancer threats like cigarette smoking. For example, with the banning of saccharin, individuals began to dwell on the possibility that the artificial sweetener could cause bladder cancer. Sadly, the majority of Americans aren't even aware that one-third of U.S. bladder cancer is directly induced by cigarette smoking.

This cancerphobia has in turn caused the diversion of limited research monies to evaluate and reevaluate food additives which have never been linked to human cancer when these funds could be more beneficially invested in a research area which shows real promise of payoff—specifically the epidemiological link between diet—general food selection, not additives—and cancer of the breast, colon, prostate, and uterus.

Further, the panic over "cancer-causing chemicals" has been divisive in creating two camps—the image of the money-grubbing industry types who do not care what is put in our foods versus the people-loving consumer activists who are dedicated to protecting all of us. The dichotomy is an absurd one. We all want our food to be safe—we also want it to be available in quantity, inexpensive, convenient, and attractive. Polarization—and that's what the Delaney Clause has created in its twenty years of existence—is not the means to that end.

One solution to this problem is the deletion of the Delaney Clause. Alternatively, the Clause could be modified—and a number of proposals have been made here. But modification would, for all practical purposes, be the same as deletion—although perhaps more politically palatable—since modification in practically any way would neutralize the Clause's main flaw—arbitrariness.

CANCER POLICY—PREVENTION, RESEARCH, EDUCATION—FOR THE FUTURE

With our increasing awareness about the role of environmental factors in the etiology of cancer, a reevaluation of our attitudes toward cancer prevention, research, and education is mandatory.

First, we should be spending our cancer dollars where they count, instead of wasting millions following false leads. For instance, an inordinate amount of time and effort has been put into intensively and repeatedly studying the artificial sweetener cyclamates, red dye #2, and other food additives, when those resources are so desperately needed in a larger area which we know is a cancer threat, but which we do not fully understand: the role of nutrition, particularly overly rich diets, and cancer. We are dealing with an estimate of 30 to 35 percent of all our country's cancer deaths being caused by poor dietary patterns and, as far as we know, zero percent being caused by food additives or pesticides. There is something desperately wrong with a cancer policy which emphasizes hypothetical risks.

Similarly, we need to look more critically at the suggestions to ban a substance like DES, which will cost the nation 800 million to one billion dollars annually—more than the National Cancer Institute's budget for a whole year—when it may be calculated that the risk from DES in beef liver is approximately equivalent to puffing one-tenth of one cigarette in a whole lifetime.

Second, we must learn to live with the concept of benefit and risk. We take risks every day. We increase our chances of death by about one in a million by smoking one and a half cigarettes, traveling fifty miles by car, two hundred and fifty miles by air—and by being a man aged sixty for twenty minutes. In our everyday lives we take a great many calculated risks. In discussing the role of alcohol and cancer, most scientists report that the most frequently asked question at the end of a talk is, "How much can I drink without having to worry about cancer?." For them, there is a perceived benefit from alcohol, and they are willing to take some risk. For some reason people appear willing to accept high personal risks (as in the case of cigarettes) but demand a much higher degree of safety for risks outside their control.

In talking about "risks" from the use of food additives, pesticides, or various occupational chemicals used in well-regulated conditions, we are not talking about tolerating the deaths or injury of X number of people a year in order for society as a whole to enjoy the benefits of those chemicals. (This *is* the case in our decision to use automobiles or airplanes; a tradeoff of life versus benefit is made.) But rather the "risk" we are talking about in using food chemicals and related substances are theoretical risks.

We cannot continue to ban food additives, pesticides, and drugs on the basis that there may hypothetically be a threat of cancer. We have got to apply some common sense to the decision-making process, taking into account how great that hypothetical risk may be—and the advantages, perhaps uniqueness, of the chemical under consideration.

Third, in discussing cancer issues, we should make a concerted effort to get our facts straight. It is inexcusable that major television networks show "special reports" on cancer without ever having their facts checked out by knowledgeable individuals. Thus we have reports telling us that "the United States is number one in cancer," and that it is additives and pesticides—hardly a word about cigarettes or diet—that are responsible for cancer deaths in our country.

Everything in America is not all wrong. Many things are very right. Our life expectancy continues to increase—and people in this country today are physically healthier than ever before. These facts make little impression on the most outspoken of the consumer advocates, whose policies and instincts seem frankly self-destructive. Their goal appears to be to undermine all the efforts of industries which are dedicated not only to their own profit motives, but to improving the quality of life in this country as well. The last decade has seen a burgeoning of antiadditive, antipesticide, antiindustry, antieverything except "natural." These individuals apparently forget that natural living includes epidemics of infectious disease, a very limited food supply, and the elimination of a wide range of technology which contributes to both our physical and mental health.

In this connection, probably the most unsettling aspect of federal regulatory activity today in the field of "chemicals" is that the word *cancer* has such a frightening connotation, that our regulators are being forced into actions not based on facts, but because of consumer pressure. We are suffering from what has been termed "political toxicology." We, as an affluent society, can handle a few of these bannings which result from political toxicology. We can do without some things. But we cannot do without everything.

Those who cry, "Cancer" at even the hint of an animal tumor are doing all of us a disfavor. They are promoting a very dangerous disease—cancerphobia. In the words of a *New England Journal of Medicine* editorial, "American cancerphobia . . . is a disease as serious to society as it is to the individual—and morally more devastating. For this state of affairs, many are to blame—not only high-pressure advertisers foment and exploit our cancerphobia, but also the well-meaning but yet baneful practices of other groups: activist, consumer organizations, politicians, and even the American Cancer Society which points direly an accusatory finger at you if you do not give money to 'cure cancer.' "

The editorial continues, "Among the guilty are the media. Because of our society's disease [cancerphobia] any news about cancer, no matter how trivial is *ipso facto* sensational. . . . So the vicious circle spirals upward and outward; cancerphobia elicits sensationalist reporting, which in turn fosters the demonology of cancer. . . . To paraphrase Justice Holmes, no one has the right to stand up in a crowded theater and shout, without adequate cause, 'Fire! Alarm! Fire'; no one, similarly, has the right to stand up in our perturbed and restless society and cry, without adequate cause, 'Cancer! Alarm! Cancer!' "

In conclusion, our "war" on cancer might receive a significant boost if we now reevaluated our concept of "cancer-causing agents," giving more attention to factors which are known to threaten our health, and less to those which "could" or "might" be involved in human carcinogenesis. This is not to say, however, that we would benefit from a complete freedom of federal, state, and local regulations with regard to the status of chemicals in the environment. Both in and out of the cancer field there have been chemical tragedies (for example, in 1973, the inclusion of a fire retardant containing a toxic industrial chemical—PBB's—in animal feed in Michigan which poisoned hundreds of thousands of farm animals and produced a wide range of illness and complaints among those who ate PBB-contaminated animal products). But a more rational, less emotionally directed approach to the regulation of carcinogens, taking preventive and remedial action where such is needed, but avoiding overreactions which lead to unwarranted bannings or restrictions—is the answer for the future.

CANCER: YESTERDAY, TODAY, AND TOMORROW

In 1900, the leading causes of death in this country were heart diseases, tuberculosis, pneumonia, and influenza. In 1978 the leading causes are heart disease, cancer, and stroke.

Will the disease patterns change drastically in the next 75 or 100 years? Will cancer fade as a health problem in the same way TB, pneumonia, and influenza did?

It is very possible that it will, but probably not (the best intentions of the American Cancer Society notwithstanding) within our lifetime. For those of us living in the latter part of the twentieth century, cancer will likely remain one of the two most serious health risks.[3] The same statement would have been made in 1940 when cancer was also the leading cause of death. But the major difference is that today, unlike thirty or forty years ago, we can do something to alter our risks. We have some personal ammunition to use against the threat of cancer. We have some potential for influencing our own fate.

3. Fortunately, at least two of the recommendations made here for avoiding cancer, giving up tobacco and modifying your diet, will also drastically reduce your odds on becoming a victim of the number-one killer, heart disease.

APPENDIX I

TIPS FOR KICKING THE CIGARETTE HABIT

"The fixity of a habit is generally in direct proportion to its absurdity."

Marcel Proust

You have a number of choices on *how* you are going to give up cigarette smoking once the decision is made. It does not matter how you do it, but you must give up cigarettes if you are to reduce your odds on developing cancer of the lung, oral cavity, and bladder and possibly other sites (as well as heart disease, stroke, emphysema, and other diseases). If one approach doesn't work, try another.

Conditioning

You may have heard of "shock treatments" for eliminating your desire to smoke. The idea here is to associate smoking with unpleasant feelings. Some require smokers to face a smoke-blowing machine, giving them electric shocks as they light up. Others require you to smoke until you vomit. Some show movies, slides, horrifying illustrations of the internal effects of tobacco—and then add an electric shock to emphasize it. Still others try all of these.

For many people, conditioning programs have helped. For some people, these programs make them more nervous, causing them to smoke more. Follow-up studies of those using the conditioning technique to kick the habit show a median success rate of about 10 to 15 percent after six months.

Hypnosis

In posthypnotic suggestion, a therapist might plant the notion that cigarettes will taste bad, cause you harm, cause you to die a premature, painful death. The long term success rates of hypnotic treatments seem to be between 20 and 40 percent.

Group Counseling

You might try joining a weekly group of smokers with intentions similar to yours. Participants in these groups (for example, those organized by Smokenders, a nationally successful group) gather to discuss smoking habits and problems in quitting, offer support and hints to each other. The group leader is often an ex-smoker, and has his or her own "how to quit" story to tell.

The success rates here depend on the type of group. Generally about half of the participants have given up smoking by the end of the four to eight weeks of meetings. Followup reports indicate the rate levels off at about 20 percent after a year.

A particularly effective program for assistance in giving up smoking has been developed by a Seventh Day Adventist clergyman, E. J. Folkenberg. His program revolves around one- to two-hour meetings of twenty to one hundred smokers for five consecutive days. During the meetings participants see films, hear lectures on the hazards of smoking, the benefits of quitting, and are encouraged to follow a rigorous daily program of physical exercise, breathing deeply, taking hot and cold showers, drinking lots of water, and abstaining from alcohol. Median success rates here have been about 60 percent, followup studies showing that about 40 percent are off cigarettes after three months, 30 percent after six months, 20 percent after one year.

Drugs

Your phyician may offer you a drug, possibly a mild tranquilizer, to help you withdraw from the addictive chemicals in cigarettes. He might also be able to help head off the possible problem of weight gain at the very beginning. Giving up smoking need not necessarily mean that you will put on weight. Often ex-smokers do put on a few pounds—primarily because food tastes so much better that they eat more of it. But by using carrots, celery, and other low-calorie food to take care of the desire to "have something in your mouth" (for some people, the plastic cigarettes, or a sturdy pen, do the job here), and by cutting back on salt you can both keep your current weight and give up cigarettes.

Don't fall into the "Well, it's unhealthy to be fat, so I might as well smoke and keep slim" trap. The problems are on two very different levels. Cigarettes increase by manyfold your chances of developing many types of cancer. Being overweight—or even obese—is not desirable but when it does occur in the course of giving up smoking, it is usually temporary, and the problem can be readily dealt with.

SOME SPECIFICS

Dr. Donald T. Fredrickson's "How to Stop Smoking Plan"
(Reprinted with the permission of Dr. Fredrickson and the American Heart Association)

STEP 1 FIRST WEEK

Before you begin a smoking withdrawal program you should do some serious thinking about sincerity of purpose and readiness to follow through. Here are some ground rules:

1. List several reasons for giving up smoking that are intensely personal, that have meaning for you.

2. Find someone who is interested in following a smoking withdrawal program with you and willing to compare notes with you as you follow the program.

3. Agree that you will follow all instructions in your program to the letter.

4. Determine that you will approach your smoking withdrawal in a positive way and not with grim determination.

Are you ready to work with us now? If so, proceed with Step 1.

1. Your first job is to build motivation. From your list of reasons for giving up smoking select the most important reason; that is, the one that will turn you on and keep you moving. Write it down.

2. Begin to think about how you should change your behavior if you wish to succeed. Write these ideas down.

3. Adopt a positive attitude. What has been your attitude before? Describe. Indicate what attitude you are going to have now.

4. Develop a Cigarette Tally of your smoking behavior. Using the following model, draw up a chart on an 8½″ x 11″ sheet of paper. This paper will be used for recording information about each cigarette you smoke during the day, including Time, Occasion, Feeling, and Value—on a scale of 1 (most important) to 5 (least important).

CIGARETTE TALLY
Date October 1

	Time	Occasion	Feeling	Value
1.	8:00 A.M.	rising	depressed	1
2.				
3.				
4.				

a. Fold the Cigarette Tally sheet lengthwise twice; wrap it around your cigarette pack; and secure the package with two rubber bands.

b. Carry your pack where you normally do and continue smoking as you have done before.

c. Every time you take a cigarette, unwrap the Tally Sheet, and fill in the appropriate information.

STEP 2 SECOND WEEK

Have you cut down on your smoking as a result of the wrapping and recording procedure? Which cigarettes were most important to you?

Most people find that the wrapping technique makes it impossible for them to smoke automatically. In addition, tallying related activities helps them to see the powerful associations that they have linked with the smoking act. They then realize that smoking is not an addiction but a habit which they have taught themselves by constantly associating actions with feelings and activities. Once they realize this they can see their way clear to the conclusion that they can reverse the process they themselves began—they can retrain themselves.

Instructions

1. Continue with your smoking record.

2. Write down the important reasons why you want to stop smoking.

3. Carry your cigarettes in a different place. If you normally carry them in one pocket, switch to another. But, whatever you do, make it a little more difficult to reach for your pack.

4. Never buy a carton of cigarettes from here on. Instead, buy one pack at a time.

5. Switch your brand at least twice during the week.

6. Do not carry matches or a lighter from now on.

7. Begin a gradual program of reduction.

a. Each morning jot down the number of cigarettes you think you can manage on for the day. at night write down how many cigarettes you actually smoked.

b. Reduce the number of cigarettes you smoke each day in any way you wish; that is, aim for eliminating the most important cigarettes or the least important. It is up to you to decide what plan will work for you.

STEP 3 THIRD WEEK

Now you are going to take a Smoker's Test, but first I'd like you to look over the smoking record that you've been keeping for the past two weeks. Can you identify those circumstances under which you smoked heavily? Which were the most important cigarettes in your daily routine?

Some people find that if they go after the toughest cigarettes first, the others take care of themselves. Others prefer to go after the 3's, 4's, and 5's—those that aren't quite that important. Once they've eliminated those, they're ready to tackle the tough ones. No two smokers smoke for the same reasons. This is simply a reflection of the fact that no two people are quite alike. So, now let's find out some of the reasons why you smoke!

Smoker's Test

The test you are about to take will help you to identify the type of smoker you are, and some of the important reasons why you continue to smoke. It was designed by Daniel Horn, Ph.D., Director of the National Clearinghouse for Smoking and Health, Public Health Service, and is based on a model developed by Silvan Tomkins, Ph.D.

Why Do You Smoke?

Here are some statements made by people to describe what they get out of smoking cigarettes. HOW OFTEN do you feel this way when smoking them? Circle one number of each statement.
Important: Answer every question.

STEP 4 FOURTH WEEK

What has been most helpful to you when the urge to smoke came upon you? As you continue your withdrawal program this week, here are some suggestions given by former smokers:

1. Walking or exercise helps. A change in activity patterns and an increase in physical exercise relieve you of excess nervousness.

2. Avoid some of the closer associations developed in smoking. Substitute other activities for ones you associate with smoking; e.g., TV, coffee. These will not need to be permanent substitutions.

3. Decide that you are not going to let the "tail wag the dog"; that is, each time you reach for a cigarette think, "I am not going to allow myself to be a Pavlovian creature with a conditioned response."

4. Substitute opposite gestures. For example, instead of reaching for a cigarette, move something away from you.

STEP 5 FIFTH WEEK

Craving

Some people find that during withdrawal they gain weight. If this is your problem, here are some hints about what to do:

1. Get a bit of extra exercise to burn up those extra calories.

2. Reach for low calorie snack foods.

During withdrawal, smokers complain of a variety of symptoms including tightness in the chest, being out of breath, dizziness, perspiring. There is no real physical basis for these symptoms and most of them subside within a few weeks. Usually the symptoms reflect anxiety. The body is learning a new way to deal with fear and tension and expresses itself in these ways. Of course, if serious symptoms persist, you should see your doctor.

Addiction vs. Habit

The reason that you have been able to work on your own smoking cure is related to the fact that smoking is a habit, not an addiction.

Addiction refers to a physical or chemical change within the body that cues you to do something. While smoking may have brought damage to your physical health and well being and the continued process can trigger chain effects of disease, it is not a chemical addiction. It is a habit—a form of learned behavior you have trained yourself in. That is the reason you can learn to be a nonsmoker. And this is why thousands of smokers each year train themselves to be nonsmokers.

Have you found yourself thinking about yourself as a nonsmoker at this point? A famous chemist named Emile Coue once said that "When your imagination is working in one direction and your willpower in another, your imagination always wins the day."

Once you begin to change your true feeling about cigarettes and what they mean in your life, so that your ideas are clear and match your will to stop, your chances of success increase. With this idea in mind you cannot be discouraged. Even if you didn't make it this time, just crawl right back on the wagon!

Remember the Ingredients of Success:

1. Find a motive or reason for stopping.
2. Change your behavior.
3. Change your attitude.

A positive attitude—a feeling that you are giving yourself a gift will be most helpful. Consider the benefits of withdrawal—getting a habit under control, a renewed feeling of self-confidence, the reduced risk of being stricken and crippled at midlife by one of the chronic diseases associated with smoking: emphysema, bronchitis, cancer, heart disease.

 American Heart Association
7320 Greenville Avenue
Dallas, Texas 75231

© Reprinted with permission American Heart Association.

	always	frequently	occasionally	seldom	never
A. I smoke cigarettes in order to keep myself from slowing down.	5	4	3	2	1
B. Handling a cigarette is part of the enjoyment of smoking it.	5	4	3	2	1
C. Smoking cigarettes is pleasant and relaxing.	5	4	3	2	1
D. I light up a cigarette when I feel angry about something.	5	4	3	2	1
E. When I have run out of cigarettes I find it almost unbearable until I can get them.	5	4	3	2	1
F. I smoke cigarettes automatically without even being aware of it.	5	4	3	2	1
G. I smoke cigarettes to stimulate me, to perk myself up.	5	4	3	2	1
H. Part of the enjoyment of smoking a cigarette comes from the steps I take to light up.	5	4	3	2	1
I. I find cigarettes pleasurable.	5	4	3	2	1
J. When I feel uncomfortable or upset about something, I light up a cigarette.	5	4	3	2	1
K. I am very much aware of the fact when I am not smoking a cigarette.	5	4	3	2	1
L. I light up a cigarette without realizing I still have one burning in the ashtray.	5	4	3	2	1
M. I smoke cigarettes to give me a "lift."	5	4	3	2	1
N. When I smoke a cigarette, part of the enjoyment is watching the smoke as I exhale it.	5	4	3	2	1

O. I want a cigarette most when I am comfortable and relaxed.	5	4	3	2	1
P. When I feel "blue" or want to take my mind off cares and worries, I smoke cigarettes.	5	4	3	2	1
Q. I get a real gnawing hunger for a cigarette when I haven't smoked for a while.	5	4	3	2	1
R. I've found a cigarette in my mouth and didn't remember putting it there.	5	4	3	2	1

SCORE CARD

$$\frac{}{A} + \frac{}{G} + \frac{}{M} = \text{Stimulation}$$

$$\frac{}{B} + \frac{}{H} + \frac{}{N} = \text{Handling}$$

$$\frac{}{C} + \frac{}{I} + \frac{}{O} = \text{Pleasurable Relaxation}$$

$$\frac{}{D} + \frac{}{J} + \frac{}{P} = \text{Crutch: Tension Reduction}$$

$$\frac{}{E} + \frac{}{K} + \frac{}{Q} = \text{Craving: Psychological Addiction}$$

$$\frac{}{F} + \frac{}{L} + \frac{}{R} = \text{Habit - Reflex}$$

When you have completed the test, score yourself:

1. Take the numbers on the first line and add across; that is add the numbers for **A**, **G**, and **M** and put the total in the last column.

2. Follow the same procedure for each line.

Scores can vary from 3 to 15. Any score 11 and above is high; any score 7 and below is low.

Instructions

1. Continue all earlier instructions.

2. But now plan a 24-hour period when you will try to go without smoking entirely.

3. Put your resolution into practice.

4. *Write a description of what happened during your "no smoking" period.*

APPENDIX II

PRUDENT EATING MADE ELEGANT

"Habit is habit, and not to be flung out the window by any man, but coaxed downstairs, a step at a time."

Mark Twain

Many of the low cholesterol, low fat, diets look very grim and unappetizing: grated peel of one orange, ¼ cup of rinsed cottage cheese, three crackers and black coffee seem to be the more commonly included items.

These types of menus overlook the fact that eating is one of the primary pleasures of life and there is no reason to sacrifice elegance and taste in favor of prudence.

Below are some examples on how you can keep your fat and cholesterol levels low and still enjoy eating. The suggestions below are of a general nature—not right for the calorie needs of everyone.

FACTS FOR FIGHTING CANCER

In planning prudent meals follow the three basic rules:

   —limit your cholesterol intake to under 300 mg. a day
   —limit your intake of all fat to 80 grams a day, preferably below that,

making sure that no more than thirty to thirty-five percent of your
total calories are contributed by fats.

—in choosing which types of fatty foods to include, stress those which
are polyunsaturated fats, skimp significantly on those high in saturated fat.

Cholesterol and Food

High cholesterol foods include brains, livers, sweetbreads, hearts, egg
yolk, untrimmed beef, butter, cheeses, and other dairy products, lard and
other animal fat.

Medium and low cholesterol foods include chicken, turkey, veal, fish,
and cottage cheese. There is no cholesterol in egg whites, margarine and
other vegetable fats, skim milk, and foods of plant origin such as fruits,
vegetables, cereals, legumes, nuts or oils.

Use Table 1 in planning your menus in the future. Remember, 300 mg.
is the maximum per day. If possible, keep your cholesterol intake well
below this. For the sake of comparison, use Table 1 to estimate how much
cholesterol you took in during yesterday's meals. This will give you an idea
of how much cutting back you'll have to do.

Fat

High fat foods include untrimmed beef, frankfurters, pies, frosted chocolate cakes, salad and cooking oils. Chicken and veal have medium
amounts of fats—and swordfish and white enriched breads have low
amounts.

Most vegetables and fruits, cereals, rice, noodles and angel food cake
are among the foods with only traces of fat. Use Table 2 to calculate how
much fat you consumed yesterday. Again, the goal is to limit your fat consumption to thirty to thirty-five percent of total daily calories. Given that
fats contribute 9 calories per gram, you can calculate the number of grams
this would allow. For example if you consume 1800 calories a day, some
600 calories (maximum) could be fat, the equivalent of about 75 grams.
Eighty grams of fat might be considered the upper limit for most average,
moderately active adults.

TABLE 1

Approximate Cholesterol Content of Selected Foods

		MG. CHOLESTEROL
	PORTION	PER EDIBLE PORTION
Beef, cooked and trimmed	4 oz.	102
Brains, cooked, no fat added	3 oz.	2,674
Butter	1 pat	20
Cheese: Cheddar, processed	1 oz.	45
Cottage, creamed	1 cup	23
Cream	1 oz.	36
Spreads, cheese foods	1 oz.	39
Chicken, Turkey, cooked	4 oz.	85
Cream: Light	1 tbsp.	11
Half-and-half	1 tbsp.	6
Eggs: Whole	1 med.	235
Yolk	1 med.	235
White	1 med.	0
Fish: Lean and medium fat	4 oz.	79
Fried	4 oz.	90
Gefilte fish	3 oz.	54
Ham, cooked and trimmed	4 oz.	102
Ice cream	1 scoop	43
Kidney	3 oz.	298
Lamb, cooked and trimmed	4 oz.	102
Liver	3 oz.	213
All-vegetable margarine	1 pat	0
Mayonnaise	1 tbsp.	8
Milk: Whole	1 cup	27
Skim	1 cup	0
Pork, cooked and trimmed	4 oz.	102
Shellfish (clams, crab, lobster, mussells, shrimp), cooked	4 oz.	170
Sweetbreads	3 oz.	249
Tongue: Cooked fresh	3 oz.	119
Cooked smoked	3 oz.	179
Veal, cooked and trimmed	4 oz.	102

Note: Cholesterol is not present in foods of plant origin such as fruits, vegetables, cereal grains, legumes, nuts, or oils.

SOURCE: By permission of the Upjohn Company, Kalamazoo, Michigan, *Scope Manual of Nutrition*, Michael Latham *et al.*

TABLE 2

Fat Values of the Edible Part of Foods [a]

FOOD	APPROX. MEASURE	WEIGHT (GRAMS)	Fat [b] (TOTAL LIPID) GRAMS	Fatty Acids [b] SATU- RATED GRAMS	UNSATU- RATED GRAMS
Milk, Cream, Cheese: Related Products					
Milk, cow's					
Fluid, whole (3.7% fat)	1 cup	244	9	5	2
Fluid, nonfat (skim)	1 cup	246	trace	–	–
Cheese:					
Cheddar	1 oz.	28	9	5	3
Cottage creamed	1 cup	225	10	5	2
Ice cream, vanilla	1 scoop	71	9	5	3
Eggs					
Raw, whole	1 med.	50	6	2	3
Meat, Poultry, Fish, Shellfish, Related Products					
Beef, cooked:					
Rump roast: choice grade					
Lean and fat	4 oz.	113	21	10	11
Lean only	4 oz.	113	6	3	3
(visible fat removed at table)					
Sirloin steak, choice grade, broiled					
Lean and fat	4 oz.	113	32	16	16
Lean only	4 oz.	113	5	2	2
(visible fat removed at table)					
Hamburger, broiled					
Regular grind	3 oz.	85	17	9	8
Ground round	3 oz.	85	13	6	5
Pork, cooked:					
Ham, baked					
Lean and fat	4 oz.	113	19	8	11
Lean only	4 oz.	113	7	3	4
(visible fat removed at table)					
Roast Pork					
Lean only	4 oz.	113	8	4	3
(visible fat removed at table)					
Lamb, cooked:					
Roast leg, choice grade	4 oz.	113	14	8	5
Veal, cooked:					
Cutlet, medium fat	3 oz.	85	13	6	5
Chicken, cooked:					
Fryer, ¼ whole, med.		85	10	3	6
Fish, cooked:					
Swordfish, broiled	3½ oz.	100	6	–	–

			Fat [b]	Fatty Acids [b]	
			(TOTAL	SATU-	UNSATU-
	APPROX.	WEIGHT	LIPID)	RATED	RATED
FOOD	MEASURE	(GRAMS)	GRAMS	GRAMS	GRAMS
Tuna, packed in oil	½ cup	115	9	3	4
Shrimp	4 oz.	113	1	–	–
Bacon, broiled or fried	2 slices	14	7	2	5
Frankfurter, cooked	1 med.	51	14	–	–
Liver, calf, broiled	4 oz.	113	7	–	–
Vegetables and Vegetable Products					
Asparagus, cooked	1 cup	181	trace	–	–
Beans:					
Lima, cooked	1 cup	166	trace	–	–
Snap, green, cooked	1 cup	125	trace	–	–
Baked, with tomato,					
molasses	1 cup	187	8	2	2
Beets, cooked	1 cup	167	trace	–	–
Broccoli, cooked	1 cup	164	1	–	–
Cabbage:					
Coleslaw, raw	1 cup	120	9	1	7
Cooked	1 cup	146	trace	–	–
Carrots, cooked, diced	1 cup	160	trace	–	–
Cauliflower, cooked	1 cup	125	trace	–	–
Celery, raw	1 stalk	40	trace	–	–
Corn, sweet					
Cooked	1 ear	100	1	–	–
Canned	1 cup	169	2	–	–
Cucumbers, raw, whole	1 small	100	trace	–	–
Lettuce, leaf	1 med.	10	trace	–	–
Mushrooms, canned	1 cup	161	trace	–	–
Onions, cooked	1 cup	197	trace	–	–
Parsnips, cooked	1 cup	211	1	–	–
Peas, cooked	1 cup	160	1	–	–
Peppers, sweet, green	1 shell	62	trace	–	–
Potatoes, medium:					
Baked, peeled	1 potato	99	trace	–	–
Peeled, boiled	1 potato	122	trace	–	–
French-fried	10 pieces	57	8	2	6
Mashed with milk and					
margarine	1 cup	195	8	4	3
Potato chips	10 med.	20	8	2	6
Tomatoes, raw	1 med.	120	trace	–	–
Turnips, cooked, diced	1 cup	196	trace	–	–
Fruits and Fruit Products					
Apples, raw	1 med.	150	1	–	–

FOOD	APPROX. MEASURE	WEIGHT (GRAMS)	Fat[b] (TOTAL LIPID) GRAMS	Fatty Acids[b] SATU- RATED GRAMS	UNSATU- RATED GRAMS
Avocados, raw, cubed	¼ cup	36	6	1	4
Bananas	1 med.	150	trace	–	–
Cantaloupe	½ med.	385	trace	–	–
Cherries, raw, sweet	1 cup	130	1	–	–
Cranberry juice	1 cup	250	trace	–	–
Fruit cocktail, canned	1 cup	229	trace	–	–
Grapefruit juice, fresh	1 cup	246	trace	–	–
Lemon	1 med.	106	trace	–	–
Orange juice, fresh or canned, unsweetened	1 cup	249	trace	–	–
Strawberries, raw	1 cup	144	1	–	–
Grain Products					
Breads, rolls, etc.					
Biscuit, baking powder (2½″ diam.)	1 biscuit	38	6	2	4
Corn muffin .	1 muffin	48	5	2	2
White bread, enriched	1 slice	23	1	–	–
Whole wheat bread	1 slice	23	1	–	–
Rye bread, light	1 slice	23	trace	–	–
Plain enriched roll	1 med.	38	2	trace	trace
Hard roll	1 med.	52	2	trace	trace
Sweet roll	1 med.	55	5	1	trace
Cakes:					
Angel food,	1 2″ sec.	40	trace	–	–
Chocolate, (chocolate frosting)	1 2″ sec.	120	15	6	8
Fruitcake, dark	2″ sq.	30	5	–	–
Cupcake, plain	1 med.	60	7	1	3
Pound cake	1 slice	30	6	2	3
Doughnuts (cake type)	1 med.	32	6	1	4
Cereals (prepared):					
Bran flakes (40%)	1 cup	38	1	–	–
Corn flakes	1 cup	28	trace	–	–
Corn, wheat, rice flakes	1 cup	22	trace	–	–
Puffed wheat	1 cup	14	trace	–	–
Rice Krispies	1 cup	28	trace	–	–
Shredded wheat	1 biscuit	28	1	–	–
Wheat flakes	1 cup	28	trace	–	–
Cereal Products:					
Macaroni, enr., cooked	1 cup	140	1	–	–
Noodles, egg, cooked	1 cup	160	2	–	–

			Fat [b]	*Fatty Acids* [b]	
			(TOTAL	SATU-	UNSATU-
	APPROX.	WEIGHT	LIPID)	RATED	RATED
FOOD	MEASURE	(GRAMS)	GRAMS	GRAMS	GRAMS
Cereal Products (*cont.*)					
Rice, white, enriched,					
cooked	1 cup	193	trace	–	–
Spaghetti, enr., cooked	1 cup	160	1	–	–
Pies					
Fruit	$1/7$ cut	135	15	4	10
Custard	$1/7$ cut	130	14	5	9
Lemon Meringue	$1/7$ cut	120	12	4	8
Mince	$1/7$ cut	135	16	4	11
Pumpkin	$1/7$ cut	130	15	5	8
Fats and Oils					
Butter	1 pat	7	6	3	2
Margarine	1 pat	7	6	1	4
Cooking Fats:					
Lard	1 tbsp.	15	14	5	7
Vegetable fats	1 tbsp.	13	12	3	9
Salad Dressings:					
Commercial, mayonnaise					
type	1 tbsp.	15	6	1	4
French	1 tbsp.	15	7	1	4
Mayonnaise	1 tbsp.	15	11	2	9
Salad or Cooking Oils:					
Corn	1 tbsp.	14	14	1	11
Cottonseed	1 tbsp.	14	14	4	10
Olive	1 tbsp.	14	14	2	12
Safflower	1 tbsp.	14	14	1	12
Soybean	1 tbsp.	14	14	2	10
Sugars and Sweets					
Chocolate, plain	1 oz.	28	9	5	4
Honey	1 tbsp.	21	0	0	0
Jams, jellies, preserves	1 tbsp.	20	trace	–	–
Syrup	1 tbsp.	20	0	0	0
Sugar	1 tbsp.	12	0	0	0
Miscellaneous Items					
Beer (3.6% alcohol)	1 bottle	340	0	0	0
Carbonated beverage	8 oz.	240	0	0	0
Nuts:					
Peanuts, roasted	1 oz.	28	13	3	10
Peanut butter	1 tbsp.	16	7	1	6
Pizza (cheese), 5½″ pc.	1 piece	75	5	2	3
Popcorn with margarine	1 cup	28	12	3	9

FOOD	APPROX. MEASURE	WEIGHT (GRAMS)	Fat[b] (TOTAL LIPID) GRAMS	SATU-RATED GRAMS	UNSATU-RATED GRAMS
Soups, canned:					
Noodle type	1 cup	250	2	trace	2
Tomato	1 cup	245	3	–	–

[a] Prepared from "Table of Food Values," by Jelia Witschi, M.S., Harvard Nutrition Service, Department of Nutrition, 665 Huntington Avenue, Boston, Massachusetts 02115.

[b] Values rounded.

SOURCE: By permission of the Upjohn Company, Kalamazoo, Michigan, *Scope Manual of Nutrition*, Appendix B (F. S. Stare, *et al.*)

Saturated versus Polyunsaturated Fats

Choose more foods from the "polyunsaturated and monounsaturated" columns, many fewer from the "saturated" fat column (see Table 3).

TABLE 3
Foods According to Types of Fats

PREDOMINANTLY SATURATED FATS	PREDOMINANTLY POLYUNSATURATED FATS	PREDOMINANTLY MONOUNSATURATED FATS
Beef, veal, lamb, pork	Corn, cottonseed, safflower, soybean oils	Olive oil
Eggs		Olives
Whole milk	Margarines containing	Avocados
Whole-milk cheese	substantial amounts	Cashew nuts
Cream (sweet or sour)	of the above in	
Ice cream	liquid form	
Butter	Fish	
Some margarines	Mayonnaise, salad	
Lard	dressing	
Hydrogenated short-enings	Walnuts, filberts, pecans, almonds,	
Chocolate	peanuts	
Coconut	Peanut butter	
Coconut oil	Products made using	
Cakes, pastries	the above	
Cookies, gravy, sauces, and snack foods made from the above		

Prudent Meal Planning

There are ways to stay below the 300 mg. of cholesterol, 80 gr. of fat limit. When you next go shopping, stock up on low-fat "imitation" products: diet margarine, low fat mayonnaise, low-fat cheeses, PAM (a vegetable oil based spray which allows you to "fry" without oil)—and, of course, egg substitutes. Fill your basket with the fruits and vegetables of the season, and round out your selection with frozen and canned products. Buy a variety of cereals—bran is fine, but eating just that can prove rather uninteresting. Try a number of enriched, fortified cereals. Pick up some plain, enriched white rice, and try some of the many seasoned and flavored rices now available.

In addition to shopping at your supermarket, stop in at a large bookstore and get some "prudent" cookbooks, for example, *The Prudent Diet* (David White, publisher) by Bennett and Simon. Write to the American Heart Association (44 East Twenty-third Street, New York 10010) and ask them to send you recipes for fat-controlled, low cholesterol meals.

Then add a bit of your imagination—and you are ready to eat prudently.

SOME EXAMPLES

Your own taste, budget, and calorie restrictions will dictate what you do eat and how you maintain the "300–80 limit." But here are just three examples of nutritious, delicious meals—well within those limits.

Example #1

Breakfast:　2 slices day-old bread

2 ounces of Second Nature, Egg Beaters, or some other egg substitute

Teaspoon of vanilla

A few dashes of cinnamon

3 ounces of orange juice

4 ounces of skim milk

Diet "imitation" margarine

Coffee or tea, plain

(Soak the bread in the mixture of egg substitute, vanilla, and cinnamon. Melt one-half teaspoon of corn-oil based marga-

rine [the half-calorie margarines won't do here in cooking].
Quickly brown the bread. Serve with a sprinkle of sugar)

Lunch: Sliced tomato
Sliced cucumber
4 ounces of chicken or fish
Diet soda,[1] tea, or coffee

Dinner: Veal cutlet (3 ounces)
2 tablespoons vegetable oil
2 medium onions
¼ cup of water
2 tablespoons lemon juice
½ teaspoon crushed oregano
2 tablespoons chopped parsley

Cut veal into serving pieces. Heat oil in a large skillet. Add
veal; cook until brown on both sides, remove from pan. Add
onions and garlic; cook until onions are tender. Remove garlic; add veal, water, lemon juice, salt and oregano. Cover and
simmer over low heat, turning meat occasionally, until meat
is tender, about 30 minutes. Add additional water, if needed.
Serve with chopped parsley.

1 (1-pound) bunch fresh broccoli, or 1 (10-ounce) package
frozen broccoli
1 tablespoon vegetable oil
¼ teaspoon dry mustard
Salt and pepper as desired
3 tablespoons water
¼ teaspoon dill seed

If using fresh broccoli, trim and wash but do not dry. Measure oil into a saucepan or skillet with a tight-fitting cover.
Add broccoli, dry mustard, dill, salt, pepper, and water;
cover. Cook over medium to low heat about 15 minutes, or
until tender, separating frozen vegetables with a fork during
first few minutes of cooking. Shake covered pan several times
to prevent sticking. Makes 3 servings.

Baked potato with teaspoon of diet margarine
Angel food cake with fruit
Coffee, tea, glass or two of wine, etc.

1. If it is still available!

Example #2

Breakfast: *Fancy "Omelette"*
⅓ cup of freshly sliced mushrooms or
⅓ cup of sliced canned mushrooms
3 ounces of egg substitute
Parsley

If you are using fresh mushrooms, sauté them in a small amount of margarine for about 5 minutes. Drain off the excess oil and water. Heat your frying or omelette pan with a small amount of margarine. When it is just about to turn brown, pour in the egg substitute and cook at medium heat for 3 or 4 minutes, shaking the pan as it cooks. Add in the cooked or canned mushrooms on one side of the pan. Turn over the other side of the "egg" and cook for another minute or so.

Sprinkle with fresh or dehydrated parsley. Serve with toast and low-fat margarine spread.

or

Fruit Omelette
Follow the same recipe, but substitute fresh or canned apples, peaches, or pears for the mushrooms. And sprinkle a dash of sugar and cinnamon as you briefly sauté them. Remember to pour off the excess liquid before you add it to the egg substitute.

Lunch: Tunafish sandwich on white enriched bread with 2 teaspoons of artificial mayonnaise
Lettuce, tomato
Fruit
Coffee, tea, soft drink

Dinner: Fresh fish fillets
Lemon juice
MSG, garlic, pepper, salt, onion, parsley
Skimmed milk

Dip the fish fillets in a mixture of equal parts of lemon juice and water for a few minutes. Place the fillet in a vegetable-oiled baking dish and season lightly with MSG, pepper, powdered garlic. Sprinkle the fish with two tablespoons of lemon juice and one-fourth teaspoon of dill weed. Barely cover the fish with skimmed milk (make your own from powdered milk, if you like) and top each fillet with a slice of onion and a lemon slice. Sprinkle with parsley. Cover baking dish with lid or aluminum foil and bake in a moderate (325° F.) oven for about 30 minutes.

Glazed Julienne Carrots
3½ cups julienne carrot strips (1 pound)
¼ cup water
½ teaspoon salt
2 tablespoons soft margarine
3 tablespoons sugar, nutmeg, or chopped mint

Place carrots, water, and salt in saucepan. Cover and cook over low heat about 10 minutes (carrots should be firm). Add margarine and sugar. Continue cooking uncovered, stirring occasionally until carrots are tender and well-glazed. Sprinkle with nutmeg or mint. Makes 6 servings.

Example #3

Breakfast: Cereal with skim milk
Fresh, canned, or frozen fruit
4 ounces skim milk
toast, diet margarine, jam
Coffee, tea

Lunch: "No-Meat Lunch"
Large salad with dressing and/or fresh lima beans, ear of corn, or other fresh, frozen, or canned vegetable

Dinner: Quartered chicken
Egg substitute
Cornflake crumbs
Parsley, tarragon, salt, pepper
Vegetable oil

Dip chicken parts in small amount of egg substitute, then coat with cornflake crumbs which have been mixed with spices and herbs. Bake in lightly oiled pan at 350° for 50 minutes. Serve with rice and mushroom pilaf (below).

¼ cup vegetable oil
½ pound mushrooms, sliced
½ cup chopped onions
¼ cup chopped green pepper
One 1-pound can (2 cups) canned tomatoes

½ cup water
1 cup uncooked rice
Few grains pepper

Heat oil in large, deep skillet. Add mushrooms, onions, and green pepper and cook slowly until tender and lightly browned. Add tomatoes and water; bring to boil. Add rice and remaining ingredients. When mixture boils again turn heat low. Cover and cook, about 30 minutes or until rice is tender. Makes about 6 servings.

(Note: If drier rice is desired cover may be removed for last 5 minutes of cooking.)

APPENDIX III

CANCER'S SEVEN WARNING SIGNALS

Cancer's Seven Warning Signs

C hange in bowel or bladder habits
A sore that does not heal
U nusual bleeding or discharge
T hickening or lump in breast or elsewhere
I ndigestion or difficulty in swallowing
O bvious change in wart or mole
N agging cough or hoarseness

Reference Chart: Leading Cancer Sites, 1976[a]

	WARNING SIGNAL: IF YOU HAVE ONE SEE YOUR DOCTOR	SAFEGUARDS
Breast	Lump or thickening in the breast.	Annual checkup. Monthly breast self-exam.
Colon and Rectum	Change in bowel habits; bleeding.	Annual checkup including proctoscopy, especially for those over forty.
Lung	Persistent cough, or lingering respiratory ailment	Eighty percent of lung cancer would be prevented if no one smoked cigarettes.
Oral (including pharynx)	Sore that does not heal. Difficulty in swallowing.	Annual checkup.

	WARNING SIGNAL: IF YOU HAVE ONE SEE YOUR DOCTOR	SAFEGUARDS
Skin	Sore that does not heal, or change in wart or mole.	Annual checkup, avoidance of overexposure to sun.
Uterus	Unusual bleeding or discharge.	Annual checkup, including pelvic examination with Pap test.
Kidney and Bladder	Urinary difficulty, bleeding—in which case consult doctor at once.	Annual checkup with urinalysis.
Larynx	Hoarseness—difficulty in swallowing.	Annual checkup, including laryngoscopy.
Prostate	Urinary difficulty.	Annual checkup, including palpation
Stomach	Indigestion.	Annual checkup.

[a] SOURCE: American Cancer Society

SELECTED REFERENCES

GENERAL

Chapters 1, 2 and 14

Agran, L. *The Cancer Connection: And What We Can Do About It.* Boston: Houghton Mifflin Company, 1977.

American Cancer Society. *Cancer Facts and Figures.* New York, 1976.

————. *Cancer: A Manual for Practitioners.* Boston, 1968.

Anderson, D. "Familial Susceptibility to Cancer." *CA* 26:143, 1976.

Brody, J. E., and Holleb, A. I. *You Can Fight Cancer and Win.* New York: Quadrangle, 1977.

Brooks, S. M. *The Cancer Story.* Totowa, New Jersey: Littlefield, Adams and Co., 1973.

Carter, L. "Cancer and the Environment (I): A Creaky System Grinds On." *Science* 186:239, 1974.

Chiazze, L. "The Cancer Mortality Scare." *Journal of the American Medical Association* 236:2310, 1976.

Council on Agricultural Science and Technology. "The Environmental Protection Agency's Nine 'Principles' of Carcinogenicity." Report #54, January 19, 1976, Ames, Iowa.

Cowdry, E. V. *Etiology and Prevention of Cancer in Man.* New York: Appleton Century-Crofts, 1968.

Cox, T. H. "Cancer: A Statement of the Facts." Unpublished. E. I. du Pont de Nemours and Company, Wilmington, Delaware, June 1976.

Eckardt, R. "Extrapolating from Animals to Man: Carcinogenesis." *Journal of Occupational Medicine* 18:493, 1976.

Flamm, W. G. "The Need for Quantifying Risk from Exposures to Chemical Carcinogens." *Preventive Medicine* 5:4, 1976.

Fraumeni, J. F., ed. *Persons at High Risk of Cancer: An Approach To Cancer Etiology and Control.* New York: Academic Press, 1975.

Glemser, B. *Man Against Cancer.* New York: Funk and Wagnalls, 1969.

Gori, G., and Peters, J. "Etiology and Prevention of Cancer." *Preventive Medicine,* 4:239, 1975.

Higginson, J. "Chronic Toxicology—An Epidemiologist's Approach to the Problem of Carcinogenesis." *Essays in Toxicology.* New York: Academic Press, 1976.

———. "A Hazardous Society? Individual Versus Community Responsibility in Cancer Prevention." *Amer. Jour. of Pub. Health* 66:359, 1976.

Hixson, J. *The Patchwork Mouse: Politics and Intrigue in the Campaign to Conquer Cancer.* New York: Anchor Press, 1976.

Ingelfinger, F. J. "Cancer! Alarm! Cancer!" *New Eng. Jour. of Medicine* 293:1319, 1975.

Kolbye, A. "Cancer in Humans: Exposures and Responses in a Real World." Presented at the Symposium on Threshold Doses in Chemical Carcinogenesis, Heidelberg, Germany, March 25–26, 1976.

Kwalick, D. S., et al. "Cancer in New Jersey: The Problem and Solution (?)" *J. of the Medical Society of New Jersey* 73:869, 1976.

Mason, T., et al. *Atlas of Cancer Mortality for U.S. Counties: 1950–1969.* Washington, D.C., DHEW Publication #75, 780 (NIH), 1975.

"New Jersey–The Cancer State?." *J. of Medical Society of New Jersey* 73:707, 1976.

Pilgrim, I. *The Topic of Cancer.* New York: Crowell, 1974.

"The Politics of Cancer." CBS Reports special, Tuesday, June 22, 1976.

Rauscher, F. J., and Flamm, W. G. "Etiology of Cancer." Unpublished, 1976.

Raven, R., and Roe, F. *The Prevention of Cancer.* London: Buttersworth, 1967.

Schottenfeld, D., ed. *Cancer Epidemiology and Prevention.* Springfield, Illinois: Charles C. Thomas, 1975.

"Seventeen Principles about Cancer, or Something." *Lancet* editorial, March 13, 1976, p. 571.

Shimkin, M. *Science and Cancer.* Washington: U.S. Department of Health, Education and Welfare, 1973.

Shubik, P. "Interpretation of Test Results in Terms of Significance to Man." In *Carcinogenesis Testing of Chemicals,* L. Goldberg, ed. Cleveland: CRC Press, 1974.

Whelan, E. M., "Are You a High Cancer Risk?" *Cancer News,* June 1977.

———. "Cancerphobia in America." *Harper's Bazaar,* April 1977.

————. "Are You a High Cancer Risk?" *Harper's Bazaar*, February 1977.

————. "Stop the Technology." *Barron's*, November 1976.

TOBACCO

Chapter 3

Abbott, T. "The Rights of the Non-smoker." *Outlook* 94:763, 1910.

Butler, C. S. "On the Use of Tobacco in Prolonging Life." *Hygenia*, March 1928, p. 162.

Cole, P., et al. "Smoking and Cancer of the Lower Urinary Tract." *New England Journal of Medicine* 284:129, 1971.

Considine, B. "To Smoke or Not to Smoke." *Cosmopolitan*, April 1954.

"A Defense of Tobacco." *Literary Digest*, November 14, 1925, p. 88.

Diehl, H. S. *Tobacco and Your Health*. New York: McGraw-Hill, 1969.

Doll, R., and Hill, A. B. "Smoking and Carcinoma of the Lung." *British Medical Journal*, Sept. 30, 1950, p. 739.

Dungal, N. "Lung Carcinoma in Iceland." *Lancet*, August 12, 1950, p. 245.

Hammond, E. C. "Tobacco." In *Persons at High Risk of Cancer*, J. F. Fraumeni, ed. New York: Academic Press, 1975.

————. "Smoking in Relation to the Death Rates of One Million Men and Women." *National Cancer Inst. Monog.* 19:127, 1966.

Hammond, E. C., and Horn, D. "The Relationship between Human Smoking Habits and Death Rates." *Journal of the American Medical Assn.* 155:1316, 1954.

Hill, A. B., and Doll, R. "Lung Cancer and Tobacco." *British Medical Journal*, May 19, 1956, p. 1160.

Hyde, L. "Cigarette Smoking and Cancer of the Lung. Is there really any etiologic relationship?" *California Medicine* 98:313–317, 1963.

Levin, M., et al. "Cancer and Tobacco Smoking. A Preliminary Report." *Journal of the American Medical Assn.* 143:336, 1950.

Mattison, H., and Schneider, J. "The Facts about Cigarettes and Your Health." *Coronet*, May 1950.

Miller, L. M., and Monahan, J. "The Facts behind the Cigarette Controversy." *Reader's Digest*, July, 1954.

Nicholls, A. "Herba Panacea." *Canadian Med. Assn. J.*, May, 1942, p. 277.

Norr, R., "Cancer by the Carton." *Reader's Digest,* Dec. 1952.

Ochsner, A., *Smoking and Cancer.* New York: Julian Messner, 1954.

"Ochsner, A., and Debakey, Z. "Carcinoma of the Lung." *Arch. Surg.* 42:209, 1941.

————. Symposium on cancer: Primary Pulmonary Malignancy. *Surg. Gynecol. Obstet.* 68:435–451, 1939.

Pearl, R. "Tobacco and Longevity." *Science* 87:216, 1938.

Ratcliff, J., "The Growing Horror of Lung Cancer." *Reader's Digest,* March 1959, p. 107.

Redmond, D. E. "Tobacco and Cancer: The First Clinical Report, 1761." *New Eng. J. Med.* 282:18, 1971.

Riis, R., "How Harmful Are Cigarettes?" *Reader's Digest,* January 1950.

Rolleston, H. "Medical Aspects of Tobacco." *Living Age* 330:85, 1926.

Ross, W. "The Dangers of Smoking, The Benefits of Quitting." New York: American Cancer Society, 1972.

Rutstein, D. "An Open Letter to Dr. Clarence Cook Little." *Atlantic Monthly,* October 1957.

Schottenfeld, D., et al. "The Role of Alcohol and Tobacco in Multiple Primary Cancers of the Upper Digestive System, Larynx and Lung: A Prospective Study." *Prev. Med.* 3:277, 1974.

"Shall Tobacco Be Prohibited?" *Current Opinion* 70:318, 1921.

Shew, J. *Tobacco: Its History, Nature, Effects on the Body and the Mind.* New York: Fowler and Wells, 1849.

Smith, D. "My Own Private War." *Reader's Digest,* June 1973, p. 104.

Smoking and Health Now, A New Report and Summary from the Royal College of Physicians of London. London, England: Pitman Medical and Scientific Publishing Co., Ltd., 1971.

"Smoking and Health: The U.S. Decision." *Newsweek,* November 18, 1963, p. 61.

"Tobacco: Poison or Medicine." *Literary Digest,* February 22, 1913.

U.S. Department of Health, Education and Welfare. Smoking and Health. Report of the Advisory Committee to the Surgeon General of the Public Health Service. U.S. Govt. Print. Off., Washington, D.C., 1964.

U.S. Department of Health, Education and Welfare, Public Health Service. "The Health Consequences of Smoking." Washington, D.C.: U.S. Government Printing Office, 1967–1974 editions.

Waters, M. "The Man Who Wrote His Own Obituary." *Reader's Digest,* July 1966.

Werner, C. A. "The Triumph of the Cigarette." *American Mercury* 6:415, 1925.

Wynder, E., and Mabuchi, K. "Etiological and Environmental Factors." *Jour. of the Amer. Med. Assn.* 226:1546, 1973.

———. "Lung Cancer among Cigar and Pipe Smokers." *Prev. Med.* 2:529, 1972.

Wynder, E. "Etiology of Lung Cancer." *Cancer* 30:1332, 1972.

Wynder, E., and Hoffman, D. "Less Harmful Ways of Smoking." *Jour. Natl. Cancer Inst.* 48:1749, 1972.

———. "Experimental Tobacco Carcinogenesis." *Science* 162:862, 1968.

Wynder, E., and Graham, E. A. "Etiologic Factors in Bronchogenic Carcinoma with Special Reference to Industrial Exposures—Report on 857 proved cases." *AMA Arch. Ind. Hyg. Occup. Med.* 4:221, 1951.

———. "Tobacco Smoking as a Possible Etiologic Factor in Bronchiogenic Carcinoma." *Jour. of the Amer. Med. Assn.* 143:329, 1950.

Wynder, E. L., et al. "Tobacco." In *Cancer Epidemiology and Prevention,* D. Schottenfeld, ed. Springfield, Illinois: Charles C. Thomas, 1975.

———. "Lung Cancer in Women: Present and Future Trends." *Jour. Natl. Cancer Inst.* 51:391, 1973.

———. "The Epidemiology of Lung Cancer." *Jour. of the Amer. Med. Assn.* 213:2221, 1970.

———. "A Short Term Followup Study of Ex-Cigarette Smokers." *Amer. Rev. of Resp. Dis.* 96:645, 1967.

———. "Epidemiology of Persistent Cough." *Amer. Rev. Desp. Dis.* 91:679, 1965.

DIET
Chapter 4

Adams, R. "Natural Foods." *New England Journal of Medicine* 283:1058, 1970.

Adamson, R. H. "Occurrence of a Primary Living Carcinoma in a Rhesus Monkey Fed Aflatoxin B-1." *Journal of National Cancer Institute* 50:549, 1973.

Aries, V., et al. "The Effect of a Strict Vegetarian Diet on the Faecal Flora and Faecal Steroid Concentration. *J. Pathol.* 103:54, 1971.

"Bacteria and Etiology of Cancer of the Large Bowel." *Lancet,* Jan. 16, 1971.

Bennett, I., and Simon, M. *The Prudent Diet.* New York: David White, 1973.

References

Berg, J. W. "Diet." In *Persons at High Risk of Cancer,* J. F. Fraumeni, ed. New York: Academic Press, 1975.

———. "Can Nutrition Explain the Pattern of International Epidemiology of Hormone-Dependent Cancers?" *Can. Res.* 35:3345, 1975.

Berg, J. W., et al. "Dietary Hypotheses and Diet Related Research in the Etiology of Colon Cancer." *Health Services* Rep. 88:915, 1973.

Bessman, S., and Hochstein, P. "Borscht, Beets and Glutamate." *New Eng. Jour. Med.* 282:812, 1970.

Borchert, P., et al. "The Metabolism of Naturally Occurring Hepatocarcinogen Safrole." *Cancer Research* 33:575, March 1973.

Bove, F. J. *The Story of Ergot.* New York: S. Karger, 1970.

Burkitt, D. "Effect of Dietary Fibre on Stools and Transit Times and Its Role in the Causation of Disease." *Lancet,* December 30, 1972.

———. "Related Disease—Related Cause?" *Lancet* 2:1229, 1969.

Butler, W. H., and Barnes, J. M. "Toxic Effects of Groundnut Meal Containing Aflatoxin to Rats and Guinea-pigs", *Brit. Jour. Cancer* 17:699, 1964.

Campbell, T. C., et al. "Aflatoxin, M-1 in Human Urine." *Nature* 227:403, 1970.

Carroll, K., et al. "Dietary Fat and Mammary Cancer." *Canadian Med. Assn. Jour.* 98:590, 1968.

Cole, P. "Coffee Drinking and Cancer in the Lower Urinary Tract." *Lancet,* June 26, 1971, p. 1335.

Connor, W. E., and Connor, S. L. "The Key Role of Nutritional Factors in the Prevention of Coronary Heart Disease." *Preventive Medicine* 1:49, 1972.

Dunn, J. E. "Cancer Epidemiology in Populations in the U.S.—with Emphasis on Hawaii and California—and Japan." *Cancer Research* 35:3240, 1975.

"Effects of Aflatoxins on Liver." *Nutrition Reviews* 27:121, 1969.

Evans, I., and Mason, J. "Carcinogenic Activity of Bracken." *Nature* 208:91, 1965.

Evans, I., et al. "The Possible Human Hazard of the Naturally Occurring Bracken Carcinogen." *Biochemistry Journal* 124:28, 1971.

Higginson, J. "The Geographical Pathology of Primary Liver Cancer." *Cancer Research* 23:1624, 1963.

Hill, M. "Metabolic Epidemiology of Dietary Factors in Large Bowel Cancer." *Cancer Research* 35:3398, 1975.

Hill, M. J., et al. "Gut Bacteria and Aetiology of Cancer of the Breast." *Lancet,* August 28, 1971.

Hirono, I., et al. "Studies on Carcinogenic Properties of Bracken." *Jour. Natl. Cancer Inst.* 45-L79, 1970.

Hoffman, F., *Cancer and the Diet.* Baltimore: William and Wilkins, 1937.

Kenn, P., and Martin, P. "Is Aflatoxin Carcinogenic in Man?" *Tropical Geographical Medicine* 23:44, 1971.

Oiso, T., "Incidence of Stomach Cancer and Its Relation to Dietary Habits and Nutrition in Japan between 1900 and 1975." *Cancer Research* 35:3254, 1975.

Pamukcu, A. "Lymphatic Leukemia and Pulmonary Tumors in Female Swiss Mice Fed Bracken Fern." *Cancer Research* 32:1442, July 1972.

Pamukcu, A. M., et al. "Assay of Bracken Fern for Carcinogenic Activity." *Cancer Research* 30:902, 1970.

Poirer, L., and Boutwell, R. K. "Current Problems in Nutrition and Cancer." *Federation Proceedings* 35:1307, 1976.

Shamberger, R., and Frost, D. "Possible Inhibitory Effect of Selenium on Human Cancer." *Canadian Medical Assn. Journal* 100:682, 1969.

Shamberger, R. J., et al. "Antioxidants in Cereals and in Food Preservatives and Declining Gastric Cancer Mortality." *Cleveland Clinic Quarterly* 39:119, 1972.

Shils, M. "Nutrition and Cancer: Dietary Deficiency and Modifications." In *Cancer Epidemiology and Prevention,* D. Schottenfeld, ed. Springfield, Illinois: Charles C. Thomas, 1975.

Walker, A. "Diet and Cancer of the Colon." *Lancet* 1:593, 1971.

Whelan, E. M. "Diet and Breast Cancer." *Harper's Bazaar*, September 1976.

Wogan, G. N., and Pong, R. S. "Aflatoxins." *Ann. N.Y. Acad. Sci.,* 174:623, 1970.

Wolff, I. A., and Wasserman, A. E. "Nitrates, Nitrites, Nitrosamines," *Science* 177:15, 1972.

Wynder, E. L. "The Epidemiology of Large Bowel Cancer." *Cancer Research* 35:3351, 1975.

———. "Identification of Women at High Risk for Breast Cancer." *Cancer* 24:1235, 1969.

———. "Nutrition and Cancer." *Federation Proceedings* 35:1309, 1977.

———. "Overnutrition and Cancer." *Prev. Med.* 4:322, 1975.

Wynder, E. L. and Mabuchi, K. "Etiological and Preventive Aspects of Human Cancer." *Prev. Med.* 1:300, 1972.

Wynder, E. L., et al. "Etiology and Prevention of Breast Cancer." Unpublished. Paper presented at the VII International Symposium, Dusseldorf, Germany, June 18–19, 1976.

ALCOHOL

Chapter 5

International Agency for Research on Cancer: Alcohol and Cancer Report, Interim Report I, A.R.C. Lyons, France, December 1973.

Kamionkowski, M. D., and Fleshler, B. "The Role of Alcohol Intake in Esophageal Carcinoma." *Amer. Jour. Med. Sci.* 249:696, 1965.

Keller, A. Z., and Terris, M. "The Association of Alcohol and Tobacco with Cancer of the Mouth and Pharynx." *Amer. Jour. Public Health* 55:1578, 1965.

Kissin, B., and Kaley, M. *Alcohol and Cancer in the Biology of Alcoholism.* V. 3, B. Kissin and H. Begleiter, eds., New York: Plenum Press, 1974.

Kissin, B., et al. "Head and Neck Cancer in Alcoholics: The Relationship to Drinking, Smoking and Dietary Patterns." *Jour. of Amer. Med. Assn.* 224:1174, 1973.

Kuratsune, M., et al. "Test of Alcoholic Beverages and Ethanol Solutions for Carcinogenesis and Tumor Promoting Activity." *Gann* 62:395, 1971.

Larsson, L., et al. "Relationship of Plummer Vinson Disease to Cancer of the Upper Alimentary Tract in Sweden." *Cancer Research* 35:3308, 1975.

Lowenfels, A. B. "Alcohol and Cancer." *New York State Jour. Med.* 74:56, 1974.

Martinez, I. "Factors Associated with Cancer of the Esophagus, Mouth and Pharynx in Puerto Rico." *Jour. Natl. Cancer Inst.* 42:1069, 1969.

Rothman, K. J. "Alcohol." In *Persons at High Risk of Cancer*, J. F. Fraumeni, ed. New York: Academic Press, 1975.

Rothman, K. J., and Keller, A. Z. "The Effect of Joint Exposure to Alcohol and Tobacco on Risk of Cancer of the Mouth and Pharynx." *J. Chron. Dis.* 25:711, 1972.

Stenback, F., "The Tumorigenic Effect of Ethanol." *Acta Pathol. Mirobio. Scand.* 77:325, 1969.

Tuyns, A. J. "Cancer of the Oesophagus: Further Evidence of the Relation to Drinking Habits in France." *Intl. Jour. Cancer* 5:152, 1970.

U.S. Department of Health, Education and Welfare. "Alcohol and Health." Washington, D.C.: U.S. Government Printing Office, 1971 and 1974.

Vincent, R. G., and Marchetta, F. "The Relationship of the Use of Tobacco and Alcohol to Cancer of the Oral Cavity, Pharynx or Larynx." *Amer. Jour. Surg.* 106:501, 1963.

Vitale, J., and Gottlieb, L. "Alcohol and Alcohol-Related Deficiencies as Carcinogens." *Cancer Research* 35:336, 1975.

Wynder, E. L., and Bross, I. J. "A Study of Etiological Factors in Cancer of the Esophagus." *Cancer* 14:389, 1961.

Wynder, E. L., et al. "Environmental Factors in Cancer of the Upper Alimentary Tract." *Cancer* 10:470, 1957.

RADIATION
Chapter 6

Duffy, B. J., and Fitzgerald, P. J. "Thyroid Cancer in Childhood and Adolescence." *Cancer* 3:1018, 1950.

Gettler, A. "Poisoning from Drinking Radium Water." *Jour. of Amer. Med. Assn.* 100:400, 1933.

Glenn, J., et al. "Chronic Radium Poisoning in a Dial Painter." *Amer. Jour. of Roentgenology* 83:465, 1960.

Holleb, A. I. "Restoring Confidence in Mammography." *Cancer News* 31:10, 1977.

Jablon, S., "Radiation." In *Persons at High Risk of Cancer*, J. F. Fraumeni, ed. New York: Academic Press, 1975.

"Justice Outspeeds the Law." *Outlook*, June 20, 1928.

Lang, D. "A Most Valuable Accident." *New Yorker*, May 2, 1959, p. 49.

Liebow, A. "Encounter with Disaster: A Medical Diary of Hiroshima." *Yale Journal of Biology and Medicine* 38:61, 1965.

Martland, H. "The Occurrence of Malignancy in Radioactive Persons." *Amer. Jour. of Cancer* 15:2435, 1931.

Martland, H., and Humphries, R. E. "Osteogenic Sarcoma in Dial Painters Using Luminous Paint." *Arch. of Pathol.* 7:406, 1929.

———. "Occupational Poisoning in Manufacture of Luminous Watch Dials." *Jour. of Amer. Med. Assn.* 92:466, 1929.

Miller, R. W. "Radiation." In *Cancer Epidemiology and Prevention*, D. Schottenfeld, ed. Springfield, Illinois: Charles C. Thomas, 1975.

———. "Delayed Radiation Effects in Atomic-Bomb Survivors." *Science* 166:596, 1969.

"Necrosis of the Jaw among Workers Applying Luminous Paint on Watch Dials." *U.S. Labor Statistics Bureau Monthly* 21:1087, 1925.

"Radium Hangovers." *Time*, November 10, 1958, p. 62.

"Radium Victim No. 41." *Life*, December 17, 1951.

"Radium as Patent Medicine." *Jour. of Amer. Med. Assn.* 93:1397, 1932.

"Radium Poisoning." *Literary Digest*, April 16, 1932.

Simpson, C. L. "Neoplasia in Children Treated with X-rays in Infancy for Thymic Englargement." *Radiology* 64:840, 1955.

"Some Unrecognized Dangers in the Use and Handling of Radioactive Substances." *Jour. of Amer. Med. Assn.* 85:1769, 1925.

SUN

Chapter 7

Allison, S. D., and Wong, K. L. "Skin Cancer, Some Ethnic Differences." *Arch. Dermatol.* 76:737, 1957.

Becker, S. W. "Deleterious Effects of Sunlight on the Skin and Their Prevention." *GP* 21:82, 1960.

Blum, H. F. "On Hazards of Cancer from Ultraviolet Light." *Amer. Ind. Hyg. Assn. Jour.* 27:299, 1966.

————. *Carcinogenesis by Ultra Violet Light*, Princeton: Princeton University Press, 1959.

Daniels, F. "Sun Exposure and Skin Aging." *New York State Jour. Med.* 64:465, 1964.

Findlay, G. M. "Ultraviolet Light and Skin Cancer." *Lancet*, Nov. 24, 1928.

Freeman, R. G. "Carcinogenic Effects of Solar Radiation and Preventive Measures." *Cancer* 21:1114, 1968.

Haenszel, W. "Variations in Skin Cancer Incidence within the United States." In *Natl. Cancer Inst. Monog.*, F. Urbach, ed. No. 10, 1963, p. 225.

Hyde, J. N. "On the Influence of Light in the Production of Cancer of the Skin." *Amer. Jour. Med. Sci.* 131:1, 1906.

McCoy, J. "The Solar Keratoses and Cutaneous Cancer." *Arch. Derm. and Syphil.* 1:175, 1920.

Robbins, E., et al. "When Cancer is Only Skin Deep." *Today's Health*, July 1966, p. 31.

Willis, I. "Sunlight and the Skin." *Jour. of Amer. Med. Assn.* 217:1088, 1971.

DRUGS

Chapter 8

Adler, E. H., and Weisstein, B. "The Clinical Use of Stilbestrol." *Ohio State Med. Jour.* 37:945, 1941.

Bertling, M. Y., et al. "DES in Nausea and Vomiting of Pregnancy." *American Jour. of Obstet. and Gynec.* 59:461, 1950.

Blamey, R. W. "Immunosuppression and Cancer." *Lancet* 1:777, 1969.

Brody, H., and Cullen, M. "Carcinoma of the Breast Seventeen Years After Mammography with Thorotrast." *Surgery* 42:600, 1957.

da Silva Horta, J., et al. "Malignancy and Other Late Effects Following Administration of Thorotrast." *Lancet* 2:201, 1965.

Dieckmann, W. J. "Does the Administration of DES During Pregnancy Have Therapeutic Value?" *Amer. Jour. Obstet. Gynec.* 66:1062, 1953.

Fraumeni, J. F., and Miller, R. W. "Drug Induced Cancer." *Jour. Natl. Cancer Inst.* 48:1267, 1972.

Gitman, L., and Koplowitz, A. "Use of DES in Complications of Pregnancy." *New York State Med. Jour.* 50:2823, 1950.

Herbst, A., et al. "Adenocarcinoma of the Vagina: Association of Maternal Stilbestrol Therapy with Tumor Appearance in Young Women." *New Eng. Jour. Med.* 284:878, 1971.

———. "Prenatal Exposure to Stilbestrol: A Prospective Comparison of Exposed Female Offspring with Unexposed Controls." *New Eng. Jour. Med.* 292:334, 1975.

———. "Clear Cell Adenocarcinoma of the Vagina and Cervix in Girls: Analysis of 170 Registry Cases." *Amer. Jour. of Obstet. Gynec.* 119:713, 1974.

———. "Vaginal and Cervical Abnormalities after Exposure to Stilbestrol in Utero." *Obstet. and Gynec.* 40:287, 1972.

Hoover, R., and Fraumeni, J. F. "Drugs." In *Persons at High Risk of Cancer*, J. F. Fraumeni, ed. New York: Academic Press, 1975.

———. "Risk of Cancer in Renal Transplant Recipients." *Lancet* 2:55, 1973.

Hudgins, A. "Stilbestrol in Obstetrics." *Medical Times*, May 1943.

Jukes, T. H. "Estrogens in Beef Production." Unpublished, Dec. 10, 1975.

Robinson, D., and Shettles, L. B. "The Use of DES in Threatened Abortion." *Amer. Jour. Obstet. and Gynec.* 63:1330, 1952.

Ryan, K. "Cancer Risk and Estrogen Use in the Menopause." *New Eng. Jour. Med.* 293:1199, 1975.

Shubik, P. "Iatrogenic Cancer: Missed Opportunities." *Hospital Practice,* October 1974, p. 12.

———, "Medical-Iatrogenic Cancer." In *Environment and Cancer,* collection of papers presented at the 24th Annual Symposium on Fundamental Cancer Research, Baltimore: The William and Wilkins Co., 1972.

Smith, D., et al. "Association of Exogenous Estrogen and Endometrial Cancer." *New England Jour. Med.* 293:1164, 1975.

Smith, O. W., et al. "The Influence of DES on the Progress and Outcome of Pregnancy as Based on a Comparison of Treated and Untreated Primigravidas." *Amer. Jour. Obstet. and Gynec.* 58:994, 1949.

———. "DES in the Prevention and Treatment of Complications Pregnancy." *Amer. Jour. Obstet. and Gynec.* 56:821, 1948.

Ulfelder, H. "Stilbestrol, Adenosis and Adenocarcinoma." *Amer. Jour. Obstet. and Gynec.* 117:794, 1973.

———. "Current Status of the Stilbestrol-Adenosis-Carcinoma Syndrome." *Recent Prog. in Obstet. and Gynec.,* Conference, August 12–18, 1973.

"Vaginal Adenocarcinomas and Maternal Oestrogen Ingestion." *Lancet,* February 16, 1974.

Vessey, M. P. et al. "Investigation of the Possible relationship between Oral Contraceptives and Benign and Malignant Breast Disease." *Cancer* 28:395, 1971.

Weiss, N. "Risks and Benefits of Estrogen Use." *New Eng. Jour. Medicine* 293:1200, 1975.

Wynder, E. L. and Schneiderman, M. A. "Exogenous Hormones— Boon or Culprit." *Jour. Natl. Cancer Inst.* 51:729, 1973.

Ziel, H., and Finkle, W. "Increased Risk of Endometrial Carcinoma among Users of Conjugated Estrogens." 293:1167, 1975.

SEX

Chapter 9

Fraumeni, J. F., et al. "Cancer Mortality among Nuns: Role of Marital Status in Etiology of Neoplastic Disease in Women." *Jour. Natl. Cancer Inst.* 42:455, 1969.

Henderson, B. E., et al. "Sexual Factors and Pregnancy." In *Persons at*

High Risk of Cancer, J. F. Fraumeni, ed. New York: Academic Press, 1975.

Lilienfeld, A. M. "The Epidemiology of the Breast Cancer." *Cancer Research* 23:1503, 1963.

MacMahon, B., et al. "Etiology of Human Breast Cancer: A Review." *Jour. Natl. Cancer Inst.* 50:21, 1973.

Mirra, A. P., et al. "Breast Cancer in an Area of High Parity: Sao Paulo, Brazil." *Cancer Research* 31:77, 1971.

Mustacchi, P. "Ramazzini and Rigoni-Stern on Parity and Breast Cancer." *Arch. Int. Med.* 108:639, 1961.

Scotto, J., and Bailar, J. C. "Rigoni-Stern and Medical Statistics." *Jour. Hist. Med.* 24:65, 1969.

Rigoni-Stern, "Fatti statistici relativi alli malattie cancerose." *Gior Servire Prop. Path. Terap.* 2:507, 1842.

Rotkin, I. D. "Relationship of Adolescent Coitus to Cervical Cancer Risk." *Jour. of Amer. Med.* 179:486, 1962.

Smith, F. R. "Etiologic Factors in Carcinoma of the Cervix." *Amer. Jour. Obstet. Gynecol.* 21:18, 1931.

Staszewski, J. "Age at Menarche and Breast Cancer." *Jour. Natl. Cancer Inst.* 47:935, 1971.

Trichopoulos, D., et al. "Menopause and Breast Cancer Risk." *Natl. Cancer Inst.* 48:605, 1972.

Valaoras, V. G., et al. "Lactation and Reproductive Histories of Breast Cancer Patients in Greater Athens 1965–1967." *Int. Jour. Cancer* 4:350, 1969.

Wynder, E. L., et al. "Study of Environmental Factors in Carcinoma of Cervix." *Amer. Jour. Obstet. Gynec.* 68:1016, 1954.

OCCUPATION
Chapter 10

Agran, L., "Getting Cancer on the Job." *Nation*, April 12, 1975, p. 433.

Anderson, A., "The Hidden Plague" *New York Times Magazine*, October 27, 1974, p. 96.

"Asbestos Hazard." *British Jour. of Med.*, Nov. 10, 1973.

Bloch, J. B. "Angiosarcoma of the Liver Following Vinyl Chloride Exposure." *Jour. of Amer. Med. Assn.* 229:53, 1974.

Brodeur, P. "Annals of Industry: Casualties of the Workplace." *New Yorker*, Oct. 29, 1973.

————. "The Magic Mineral," *New Yorker*, Oct. 12, 1968.

Demy, N., and Adler, H. "Asbestosis and Malignancy." *Amer. Jour. Roentgenology* 100:597, 1967.

Dutton, H. "Asbestos Claim Succeeds." *Lancet*, July 25, 1970.

Eckhardt, R. *Industrial Carcinogens*. New York: Grune & Stratton, 1959.

Enterline, P. E., and Henderson, N. "Type of Asbestos and Respiratory Cancer in the Asbestos Industry." *Arch. Env. Health* 27:312, 1973.

Fraser, T. M., et al. "Occupational Cancer." *Ohio State Med. Jour.* 55:1217, 1959.

Gilson, J. C. "Asbestos Cancer: Past and Future Hazards." *Pro. Roy. Soc. Med.* 66:395, 1973.

Hueper, W. C. *Occupational Tumors and Allied Diseases*. Springfield, Illinois: Charles C. Thomas, 1942.

Kleinfeld, M., et al. "Mortality Experience in a Group of Asbestos Workers." *Arch. Env. Health* 15:177, 1967.

Lorenz, E. "Radioactivity and Lung Cancer." *Jour. Natl. Cancer Inst.* 5:1, 1944.

Merliss, R. R. "Talc Treated Rice and Japanese Stomach Cancer." *Science* 173:1141, 1971.

"More Facts on Vinyl Chloride and Cancer." *British Med. Jour.*, November 1974, p. 486.

Newhouse, M. "The Medical Risks of Exposure to Asbestos." *The Practitioner* 199:285, 1967.

Poole-Wilson, D. S. "Occupational Tumors of the Bladder." *Proc. of Royal Soc. of Med.* 53:801, 1959.

Royall, H. J. "The Health of the Public and Asbestos Usage." *Jour. Royal Inst. Public Health and Hygiene* 29:126, 1966.

Scott, T. S. *Carcinogenic and Chronic Toxic Hazards of Aromatic Amines*. Amsterdam: Elisevier Publishing, 1962.

Selikoff, I., and Hammond, E. C. "Community Effects of Nonoccupational Environmental Asbestos Exposure." *Amer. Jour. of Pub. Health* 58:1658, 1968.

Thompson, W. "The Problem of Asbestos." *Nursing Times*, Nov. 12, 1970.

"Vinyl Chloride and Cancer." *Brit. Med. Jour.*, March 30, 1974.

ADDITIVES AND PESTICIDES
Chapter 11

Abelson, P. "Chemicals and Cancer." *Science* 166:633, 1969.

Alexander, T. "The Hysteria about Food Additives." *Fortune,* March 1972.

Anderson, K. "After Cyclamates: What's Next on the FDA's Food Target List?" *Science Digest,* February 1970.

Barrons, K. *The Food in Your Future.* New York: Van Nostrand/Reinholt, 1975.

Berg, J. W. "Diet." In *Persons at High Risk of Cancer,* J. F. Fraumeni, ed. New York: Academic Press, 1975.

Bernarde, M. A. *The Chemicals We Eat.* New York: American Heritage Press, 1971.

Bickel, L. *Facing Starvation: Norman Borlaug and the Fight Against Hunger.* New York: Reader's Digest Press, 1974.

Blank, C. "The Delaney Clause: Technical Naivete and Scientific Advocacy in the Formulation of Public Health Policies." *California Law Review* 62:1084, 1974.

Bryan, G. T., and Yoshida, O. "Artificial Sweeteners as Urinary Bladder Carcinogens." *Arch. Environ. Health* 23:6, 1971.

Bryan, G. T. and Erturk, E. "Production of Mouse Urinary Bladder Carcinomas by Sodium Cyclamate." *Science* 167:996, 1970.

Council on Agricultural Science and Technology. "Hormonally Active Substances in Foods: A Safety Evaluation." Report #66, February 1977.

———. "Chlordane and Heptachlor." Report # 47, Oct. 3, 1975.

Crampton, R. F. "Problems of Food Additives, with Special Reference to Cyclamates." *Brit. Med. Bull.* 197:333, 1970.

"The Cyclamate Bandwagon." *Nature,* Oct. 25, 1969, p. 298.

Damon, G. E. "Primer on Food Additives." Department of Health, Education and Welfare Publication 74-2002, 1973.

Deutsch, R. *The Nuts among the Berries.* New York: Ballantine Books, 1961.

Epstein, S. "The Delaney Amendment." *Preventive Medicine* 2:140, 1973.

Furia, T. E. *Handbook of Food Additives.* Cleveland: The Chemical Rubber Company, 1968.

Gray, D. W. "Battle over Sweeteners Turns Bitter." *New York Times,* June 1, 1969.

Higginson, J., et al. "Nutrition and Cancer: Ingestion of Foodborn Carcingens." In *Cancer Epidemiology and Prevention,* D. Schottenfeld, ed. Springfield, Illinois: Charles C. Thomas, 1975.

Inhorn, S. L., and Meisner, L. F. "Irresponsiblity of the Cyclamate Ban." *Science* 167:1436, 1970.

Issenberg, P. "Nitrate, Nitrosamines and Cancer." *Federation Proceedings* 35:1322, 1976.

Jukes, T. H. "Diethylstilbestrol in Beef Production: What Is the Risk to Consumers?" *Preventive Medicine* 5:438, 1976.

———. "The Delaney 'Anti-Cancer' Clause." *Preventive Medicine* 2:133, 1973.

———. "Scientific Agriculture at the Crossroads." *Nutrition Today* 8:31, 1973.

———. "Fact and Fancy in Nutrition and Food Sciences." *Journal of the American Dietetic Association* 59:203, 1971.

Kermode, G. O. "Food Additives." *Scientific American* 226:315, March 1972.

Maddox, J. *The Doomsday Syndrome: An Attack on Pessimism.* New York: McGraw-Hill, 1972.

Manufacturing Chemists Association. *Food Additives: Everyday Facts.* Washington, D.C., 1973.

Miller, J. A., and Miller, E. "Carcinogens Occurring Naturally in Foods." *Federation Proceedings* 35: (6)1316, 1976.

National Academy of Sciences, "Contemporary Pest Control Practices and Prospects: The Report of the Executive Committee." Washington, D.C., 1975.

National Science Foundation. *Chemicals and Health. Report of the Panel on Chemicals and Health of the President's Science Advisory Committee,* September 1973.

Roe, F. J. "Carcinogens and Food: A Broad Assessment." *Proc. Roy. Soc. Med.* 66:23, 1973.

Shubik, P. "Potential Carcinogenicity of Food Additives and Contaminants." *Cancer Research* 35:3475, 1975.

Whelan, E. M. "The Story of Saccharin." *Across the Board,* June 1977.

———. "Natural Foods: Rip-off with a Twist." *Signature,* September 1975.

———. "Panic Over Food Additives." *Washington Post,* August 10, 1975.

———. "Healthier Than Life Itself." *New York Times,* July 23, 1975.

———. "What's Your Food IQ?," *Reader's Digest,* March 1975.

———. "Can You Separate Food Fads from Food Facts?" *Glamour,* June 1974.

————. "The If-It's-Natural-It's-Good Hoax," *Connecticut College Alumni News*, Spring 1974.

————. "How Sweet It Isn't." *National Review*, January 1974.

Whelan, E. M., and Stare, F. J. "The Panic over Food Additives." *Pediatric Basics*, January 1976.

————. *Panic in the Pantry: Food Facts, Fads and Fallacies*. New York: Atheneum, 1975.

White-Stevens, R. H. "Agriculture, America's Brightest Star, Outshines Its Quibbling Critics." Council for Environmental Balance, Louisville, Ky., 1975.

STRESS

Chapter 12

Arehart-Treichel, J. "The Mind Body Link." *Science News* 106:394, 1975.

Kowal, S. "Emotions as a Cause of Cancer." *The Psychoan. Rev.* 42:217, 1955.

LeShan, L. "Psychological States as Factors in the Development of Malignant Disease: a Critical Review." *Jour. Natl. Cancer Inst.* 22:1, 1959.

Ratcliff, J. D., "How to Avoid Harmful Stress." *Today's Health*, July 1970.

Riley, V., "Mouse Mammary Tumors: Alteration of Incidence as Apparent Function of Stress." 189:465, 1975.

Riley, V., et al. "The Role of Physiological Stress and Breast Tumor Incidence in Mice." *Proc. Amer. Assn. Can. Res.* 16:152, 1975.

Selye, H. "The Evolution of the Stress Concept." *Amer. Scientist* 61:692, 1973.

Spackman, D. "The Role of Stress in Producing Elevated Cortico-sterone Levels and Thymus Involution in Mice." *XIth International Cancer Congress* 3:382, 1974.

Spackman, D., and Riley, V. "Increased Corticosterone, a Factor in LDH Virus Induced Alterations of Immunological Responses in Mice." *Proc. Amer. Assn. Cancer Res.* 15:143, 1974.

Stein, M., et al. "Influence of Brain and Behavior on the Immune System." *Science*, Feb. 6, 1976.

Whelan, E. M. "Stress and Cancer." *Harper's Bazaar*, August 1976.

AIR POLLUTION

Chapter 13

Hammond, E. C. "Smoking Habits and Air Pollution in Relation to Lung Cancer." In *Environmental Factors in Respiratory Disease*, D. Lee, ed. New York: Academic Press, 1972.

Hoffman, D. and Wynder, E. "A Study of Air Pollution Carcinogenesis." *Cancer* 15:93, 1962.

Kuschner, M. "The Causes of Lung Cancer." *Amer. Rev. Respir. Dis.* 98:573, 1968.

Menck, H., et al. "Industrial Air Pollution: Possible Effect on Lung Cancer." *Science* 183:210, 1974.

Pike, M., et al. "Air Pollution." In *Persons at High Risk of Cancer*, J. F. Fraumeni, ed. New York: Academic Press, 1975.

Royal College of Physicians of London, *Air Pollution and Health*. London: Pitman, 1970.

Sawicki, et al. "Benzo(a)pyrene Content of the Air of American Communities." *Amer. Ind. Hyg. Assn. Jour.* 21:443, 1960.

Waller, R. E. "Bronchi and Lungs—Air Pollution." In *The Prevention of Cancer*, Raven, R., and Roe, F. J. C., London: Butterworths, 1967.

Wynder E. L., et al. "The Epidemiology of Lung Cancer, Recent Trends." *Jour. Amer. Med. Assn.* 213:2221, 1970.

Wynder, E. L., and Hoffman, D. "Carcinogens in the Air." In *Environment and Cancer*. Baltimore: The Williams and Wilkins Co., 1972.

INDEX